dramatic

changes

dramatic
changes

talking about
sexual orientation
and gender identity
with high school students
through drama

paula ressler

Heinemann
Portsmouth, NH

Heinemann
A division of Reed Elsevier Inc.
361 Hanover Street
Portsmouth, NH 03801–3912
www.heinemanndrama.com

Offices and agents throughout the world

The author and publisher wish to thank those who have generously given permission to reprint borrowed material:

"Youth Bring Gay Rights Movement to School" by David Buckel from the *Lambda Update* (Fall 1999) is reprinted courtesy of Lambda Legal Defense and Education Fund.

"Students at Risk" Comparison Fact Sheet is reprinted courtesy of Parents, Families, and Friends of Lesbians and Gays (PFLAG), Bloomington-Normal, Illinois.

"Gay/Straight Alliance Flyer" is reprinted with permission of Michael Perelman and Paula Ressler.

"Batty Boys in Babylon: Can Gay West Indians Survive the 'Boom Bye Bye' Posses?" by Peter Noel and Robert Marriott from *The Village Voice*, 38 (2). Reprinted by permission of Peter Noel.

"The Names on the Board" by Jamie Rhein from *Teaching Tolerance* (Spring 1998). Copyright © 1998 by Teaching Tolerance, Southern Poverty Law Center, Montgomery, Alabama. Reprinted by permission.

"Educators Protest Limits on Multicultural Mandate" by Paula Ressler from *LEARN* (June 1995). Reprinted courtesy of Language Educators Applying Reflection Now (LEARN).

"Anniversary Song" from the Columbia Picture *The Jolson Story* by Al Jolson and Saul Chaplin. Copyright © 1946 Mood Music Division—Shapiro, Bernstein & Co., Inc., New York. Copyright renewed. This arrangement Copyright © 2002 by Mood Music Division—Shapiro, Bernstein & Co., Inc., New York. International Copyright secured. All rights reserved. Used by permission.

"We Kiss in a Shadow" from *The King and I*. Lyrics by Oscar Hammerstein II. Music by Richard Rodgers. Copyright © 1951 by Richard Rodgers and Oscar Hammerstein II. Copyright renewed. This arrangement Copyright © 2002 by Williamson Music. Williamson Music owner of publication and allied rights throughout the world. International Copyright secured. All rights reserved. Used by permission.

Library of Congress Cataloging-in-Publication Data
Ressler, Paula.
    Dramatic changes : talking about sexual orientation and gender
identity with high school students through drama / by Paula Ressler.
        p.   cm.
Includes bibliographical references.
    ISBN 0-325-00414-5 (pbk.)
    1. Drama in education.   2. Homosexuality and education.   3. Gender identity.   4. Role playing.
I. Title: Talking about sexual orientation and gender identity with high school students through
drama.   II. Title.
    PN3171 .R472002
    306.76′6′0712—dc21   2002001576

Editor: Lisa A. Barnett
Production: Lynne Reed
Cover design: Jenny Jensen Greenleaf
Typesetter: TechBooks
Manufacturing: Steve Bernier

Printed in the United States of America on acid-free paper
06   05   04   03   02   DA   1   2   3   4   5

In memory of my son,
Shandi Stephen Free Hopkins

Contents

Acknowledgments

This book has emerged from my experiences as a mother, writer, educator, scholar, and activist for social change. The idea for the book grew from a suggestion made ten years ago by Lisa Barnett of Heinemann, after she attended a workshop I facilitated at a national conference of the American Alliance for Theatre and Education. At that time, the possibility of writing a book about addressing lesbian and gay issues through drama seemed remote. But Lisa was patient, and I kept making progress.

The book also stems from my sadness for those whose lives ended prematurely and the parents and loved ones who buried them, my hope for those who are still struggling, and my wonder at those young people who survive all the odds stacked against them and somehow even thrive.

My son, Shandi Hopkins, is at the heart of all my work. His complex, sometimes wonderful and sometimes frightening life, and now his death by suicide fuel my desire to make life easier for all young people who face seemingly insurmountable obstacles and discrimination in the world around them.

I also want to acknowledge other members of my family. Shandi's half-brother, Rafi Hopkins, whom I also consider a son and whose life I will continue to celebrate, stayed at Shandi's side through some of the roughest times. Also, his uncles David Hopkins and David Wilson, who have been so loving and supportive, and his grandmother June Hopkins, who has reached out to me in her wisdom and compassion. I am grateful for the way the whole Hopkins family came together during this tragedy. Shandi would be proud of them all.

My lover, life partner, dearest friend and companion, Becca Chase, has been with me since 1983. I feel blessed to have her and to still feel so much love. Not only is she the kindest person I know, but she is also an excellent writer and editor and through our years together has helped me to gain confidence in myself as a writer.

Another very special relative in my life today is my cousin Herta Gutfreund, who fled Vienna in 1939 at age fifteen, but whose parents and sister did not survive Hitler. She has given Becca and I much love and understanding and has helped me affirm life in the midst of terrible tragedy and loss.

I am also grateful to my sister, Joan Blaha, and her late husband, George, who became cherished friends in recent years; my nephew, Mark Fligel, and niece, Lori Kaufman, who will always be dear to me; and my cousin Claudy Ehrlich and her daughter Jane Reifer, who lovingly reached out to me and renewed long-lost family connections when I most needed them. Becca's family—Herb and Virginia Wally, her parents; her aunts Esther and Anne Vincent; and Cheryl and Ray Lougeay, her stepsister and brother-in-law—have always welcomed us as a couple and accepted us for who we are. I also want to acknowledge other courageous family members who are no longer alive—my parents, Hilda and Karl Ressler, my grandparents Dora and Mayer Alter, and my uncle Arnold Alter, all who helped raise me and who fled Central and Eastern European anti-Semitism to begin their lives again in the United States—and the rest of my extended family, many of whom died in the Holocaust.

There are so many mentors and teachers who have contributed to this book's fruition. Ellen Greer and Carolyn Treadway, and Rabbi Regina Sandler-Phillips provided invaluable emotional, intellectual, and spiritual support along the way. Bob Colby and Carol Korty, my mentors from Emerson College, believed in me at a critical time in my life and gave me rich opportunities to express myself through educational drama. I also want to give special thanks to the other highly skilled drama educators I have studied with: Gavin Bolton, Cecily O'Neill, Jonothan Neelands, Augusto Boal, theatre-in-education specialists Chris Vine and Lynne Clarke, and drama therapists Robert Landy and Sue Jennings, all of whom helped me develop appropriate frameworks for what I wanted to do with lesbian, gay, bisexual, and trans (LGBT) issues in education.

I also thank the many professors, mentors, and colleagues I worked with at New York University. My friends and mentors Berenice Fisher and her partner, Linda Marks, continually inspire me as does Irene Shigaki, who invited me to do workshops for her graduate students and has embraced LGBT issues in her multicultural work and lifelong friendship. The English Education faculty provided important guidance: Marilyn Sobelman and her husband, Aaron, who reached out to my family in important ways, as well as John Mayher, Gordon Pradl, and Harold Vine. I also thank Howard Coron, in Elementary Education at NYU, who, along with Marilyn Sobelman, sponsored the Summer Institute on Critical Social Issues in Urban Education, which I codeveloped with Becca Chase, and which provided an important research venue.

My sister doctoral students and teacher education colleagues also played a tremendous role in shaping this book through their encouragement and enthusiasm about my work, particularly Sharon Shelton-Colangelo and Bill Colangelo, Gail Verdi, and Diana-Elena and David Matsoukas. Other colleagues who gave me their support and encouragement are Sherry Gorelick at Rutgers; Tania Ramalho at SUNY Oswego; Marie Lovrod at Goddard College; and Ron Madson of the New York City Lesbian and Gay Teachers Association.

This book also owes its inspiration to the people I worked with at City-As-School High School in New York City, who taught me so much about their lives. Bob Lubetsky, my principal, for hiring me and supporting the formation of the school's gay/straight alliance; Irene Villasenor and Laila Braghan, former students who inspired the formation of the group; Michael Perelman, who co-facilitated the group with me; and my many other colleagues and students at the school.

I also want to pay tribute to four extraordinary educators who have recently died in the prime of their lives and careers and who have had a tremendous impact on my life and work and the lives of so many others—Lyn Fiol-Mata, Steven B. Schultz, B. Michael Hunter (Bert), and Bruce Jericeau. I miss all of you so much.

Finally, I want to thank all the adults and young people who have participated in my classes and workshops, whom I cannot name for reasons of confidentiality. These are the people who have made this book possible, who have struggled with their own beliefs and values at times and who were willing to confront an entrenched societal prejudice as an intrinsic aspect of their own education and professional development. I am grateful to all of you.

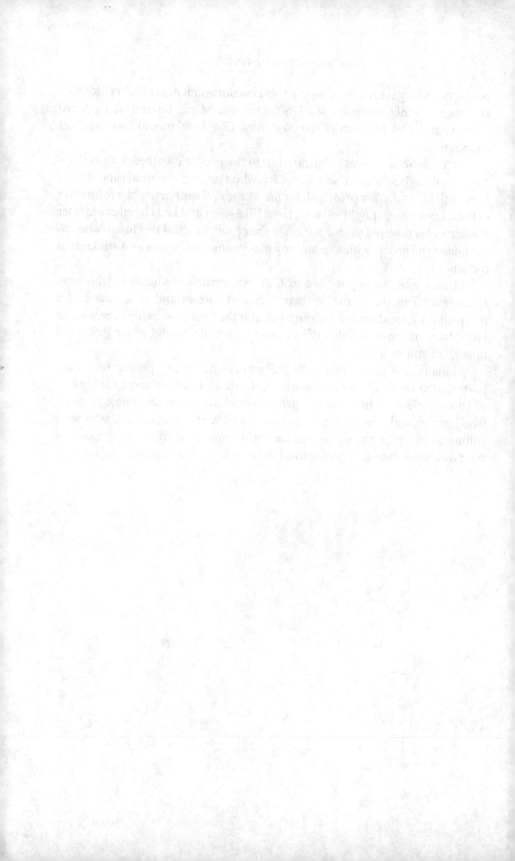

Introduction

Giving the Moment Back

I was teaching a lesson on figure drawing to a class of ninth graders. I had them doing short gesture drawings (one to two minutes) asking for volunteers from the class to be models. Only boys were getting up to model, so I asked if any girls wanted to model. This question elicited the response, "How 'bout Andy," from one boy, followed by some giggles from the rest of the class and a down-turned face from Andy. I froze, not quickly realizing just what the comment meant. It happened so fast. I overlooked it. "OK, who's next, let's go!"

After class, when the room was empty-quiet, my mind returned to the whole scenario that had just passed. I began to put things together. Craig's comment ("How 'bout Andy"), the giggles, Andy's shyness in class, his soft spoken voice, smileless face and the fact that except for Sophie, he is isolated from the class, taking comfort in the company of the one person in the class who accepts Andy for who he is—an African American gay male! . . . I began to wonder if Andy would have felt more isolated if I made a stink about it in class, if I reprimanded Craig. Maybe he would have been happy. Maybe I would have been the first teacher to finally say something. Maybe he would have dreaded it. I should have at least talked to him. Let him know the trouble I was having with it. Then at least he would have known that I was trying, thinking, that I cared. But I didn't. I blew it. I wish I had that moment back. (Richard 1994)

Richard, a white, heterosexual, male, master's preservice teacher in his early twenties, wrote this story in response to a drama workshop I conducted in one

1

of his teacher education courses on current issues in education in the spring of 1994. Like Richard, other students I have worked with also talk about not knowing how to bring up the topic of sexual orientation or how to respond when homophobia is expressed.

In his response, Richard only shares his shame about not responding in the moment. He does not address his fear of being publicly implicated in homosexuality, something that often happens when straight or gay educators intervene in homophobic name-calling. Teachers face similar risks by introducing ideas about sexual orientation and gender diversity into the curriculum or by responding positively to any references to lesbian, gay, bisexual, or trans culture that may arise in discussion. Queer educational theorist Elizabeth Ellsworth (1997) suggests that Richard's initial ignorance about what was going on was unconsciously related to his fear of being implicated in homophobia (57). Instead of feeling shame about his inability to respond to homophobia in that moment, instead of focusing on how he "blew it," she proposes that studying what happened that day, that is, thinking about why he didn't act, could teach him something more valuable (65).

Richard had not shared this story in his other teacher education classes for a variety of reasons. Most of his teacher education courses did not assign readings about sexual orientation or bring this and related topics up for discussion. I have found that unless I specifically invite students to discuss sexual orientation and gender diversity or incorporate these topics into my syllabus, most students will not risk raising them on their own, even when they have very compelling reasons to do so and significant questions to pursue.

Richard's act of writing his response demonstrates what can happen when issues about sexual and gender identity are incorporated into the teacher education curriculum, and particularly the power of drama in facilitating discussion about topics that have been suppressed in traditional education venues and therefore mired in taboo and confusion. Unlike his other teachers, the teacher of this course did assign a reading about sexual orientation (Friend 1993) and the class had had a discussion about it. But it was the follow-up drama workshop that ultimately gave Richard the permission and encouragement to risk sharing his experience. As a result of the workshop, which tapped into his emotions, he was able to bring what was unconscious and fearful to the surface, where he could entertain the possibility of responding differently.

I have received other such responses to the workshops I have facilitated. Participants talk about their fears of addressing any issues that are related to sexuality or gender. They often tell stories they do not tell in their other courses about shame and embarrassment at missed opportunities or fears of being stigmatized. They also tell stories about witnessing experienced teachers break through the barriers of silence and shame to support a student who was being harassed for being or seeming differently gendered or belonging to a sexual minority, or for being a member of a lesbian- or gay-headed family. They do not share these stories in their other classes, either.

It is widely recognized that our nation's high schools can be some of the most damaging environments for young people, particularly for those who appear to be different from the mainstream (Uribe & Harbeck 1992; Friend 1993). Students who are marginalized because of race, sex, gender, ability, sexual orientation, appearance—more likely, a combination of these factors—spend much of their time in high school just trying to survive, never mind being able to focus on learning. The consequences of not addressing these issues can be devastating for everyone.

Local teachers organizations around the country such as the Lesbian and Gay Teachers Association of New York (LGTA); social service organizations such as the Hetrick-Martin Institute; national educational organizations such as Parents, Families, and Friends of Lesbians and Gays (PFLAG), the Gay, Lesbian, and Straight Education Network (GLSEN) and Project 10; and others have been doing excellent work counteracting homophobia in educational settings across the country for a number of years, particularly emphasizing issues of safety. This book is designed both to supplement those efforts and to take that work in new and different directions. The drama workshops described in these pages reflect the work of many people and organizations. They draw upon the latest research from the fields of psychology, sociology, and education about the difficulties lesbian, gay, bisexual, trans, and questioning youth face: violent peer and family relations; high suicide rates, incidences of drug abuse, risk of contracting sexually transmitted diseases, and dropout rates; and homelessness. Participants in all antihomophobia workshops generally gain access to a wealth of information, including how homophobia, transphobia, and heterosexism pervade society; how this prejudice affects everyone; what measures people have taken to combat discrimination against sexual and gender minorities; and the roles that gay, lesbian, bisexual, and trans people have played in history and culture. It is how participants gain access and what they do with the information that distinguishes these drama workshops from other kinds of antihomophobia/transphobia work.

Inquiring into matters of sexual orientation and gender identity through drama offers a Freirian (1970/1993) approach to teaching and learning in which new knowedge is experienced rather than transmitted. Instead of being told about how sexual or gender minority youth suffer in schools, participants in a drama workshop will meet or become involved virtually and vicariously in the life of such a young person. Or they might feel the frustration of a closeted teacher who cannot meet her students' needs or the confusion of a principal who is trying to balance the concerns of students, teachers, parents, superintendent, and school board. They might have all these experiences during the course of one workshop or several.

Introduction to Terminology

Language is one of the many ways in which sexual and gender minorities are oppressed. There are probably more words with negative connotations about people who cross or live their lives on the borders of sex and gender norms than about any other group of people in society. This is true across differences of race, ethnicity, language, geography, and culture.

But at the same time that language is oppressive, it is also a place of liberation. People who identify themselves as lesbian, bisexual, gay, transsexual, transgender, or intersexual are redefining words and concepts as they struggle to situate and define themselves in a world in which they are considered other. Words and definitions in this world are continually in flux.

For this book, I define *transsexual* as referring to men and women who cross the borders of the sex they were assigned at birth, sometimes surgically and hormonally, and *transgender* as referring to people for whom gender boundaries assigned at birth eventually become blurred (Feinberg 1997), because these terms are misunderstood and are rarely used in traditional K–12 settings. In continuing to also use the more familiar terms of *gay*, or *lesbian gay*, in this book, I refer to a community that is much broader and diverse than these terms signify. I also refer to *LGBT* or *trans people*, meaning lesbian, gay, bisexual, transgender, and transsexual. When referring to sexual and gender minority youth, people often add the letter Q to the term *LGBT*, meaning youth who are questioning their sexual orientation and gender identities. Other times people use the term *LGBTQP*, incorporating people *perceived* to be gay.

Occasionally, I also use the word *queer* in the book, a term I prefer because it is more inclusive and political and reflects a more postmodern view that identities often are not fixed and are more fluid than we usually assume. The term is considered transgressive, however, and some people still consider it offensive because of its pejorative roots. Using the term *queer* is also more inclusive of intersexed people, "individuals born with anatomy or physiology which differs from cultural ideals of male and female" (ISNA 1996), some of whom see themselves as members of the transsexual/transgender community and some who do not.

Some people also reject the term *queer* as being exclusive of women, although this is less true today. The term *queer* has become so popular that it has been accepted into the academy, and many colleges and universities have courses in queer theory and departments of queer studies. I continue to experiment with language and meaning in my own work and hope that my use in this book of many terms with which people may not be familiar will help readers build a broader vocabulary for signifying sexual and gender difference and embracing diversity.

Language, Learning, and Drama

Because prejudice and social constructions of identity are formed on a deep emotional level, drama, with its strong affective component, can help people talk about and reflect upon their prejudices in ways that other classroom practices cannot. By allowing participants to step into the shoes of another, drama can compel people to challenge their assumptions and learn that what they think and what others think about sexual and gender identity is socially constructed. Working through role in a drama also helps participants gain understanding and empathy or sympathy for others. British language arts theorist Douglas Barnes (1976/1992) recognizes that sympathy is critical to learning. "Only by an act of sympathy can they bring the poem and their own lives into relation with one another . . . Unless pupils are willing to take the risk of some emotional commitment they are unlikely to learn" (87).

Drama also helps students to incorporate new knowledge into their lives. Developmental psychologist Jean Piaget (1964/1967) emphasizes that new knowledge must be linked to what students already know in order for it to be useful. The dramatic mode bridges the gap between what people already know and what they are learning. As British language arts educator John Dixon explains, "'Drama' means doing, acting things out rather than working on them in abstract in private. When possible it is the truest form of learning, for it puts knowledge and understanding to their test in action" (1975, 43).

British linguist James Britton (1982) points out that we shape our thoughts through ordinary face-to-face speech. He stresses the value of "spontaneous inventiveness" or what he calls "shaping at the point of utterance" (139), as being crucial to helping us "make sense of what is happening around us" (141). He says it is also "the language in which we first-draft most of our important ideas . . . and it's the form of language by which most strongly we influence each other" (97). This explains why writing that grows out of drama is often deeper in meaning and more detailed than other first-draft writing.

As an English teacher, some of what excites me most about working through drama is its encouragement of exploratory thought, speech, and writing. In role, people often use language they have never used, discuss topics they would not broach ordinarily, and draw upon emotions they rarely express. They may say things they believe in strongly and never had the courage to say or say things they do not believe in to help them understand opposing views. Both practices help them examine multiple aspects of a situation and construct a reality that encompasses more than just themselves and their own limited experiences. Drama therapists further explain drama's ability to do this. Stepping into role, they explain, helps us distance ourselves from our own emotions, bringing unconscious feelings and thoughts to the surface and making it easier to talk about feelings or ideas we have not previously examined (Emunah 1994; Johnson 1981; Landy 1986, 1993).

Linguists, language arts educators, and cognitive psychologists all emphasize that speaking is deeply related to thinking (Barnes 1976/1992; Britton 1982; Dixon 1975; Halliday 1989; Vygotsky 1915-1935/1978). Nevertheless, drama is not widely valued in schools as a pedagogical tool because it relies heavily on oral language. Language arts educator James Moffett (Moffett & Wagner 1973/1976), who emphasizes how "verbalization translates thought into speech" (122), points out that schools have slighted oral language because it cannot be uniformly programmed and predicted (17).

Howard Gardner (1983/1985, 1993, 1995) makes a similar point in his theory of multiple intelligences. He shows that this culture values only certain forms of intelligence—verbal-linguistic intelligence and logical-mathematical—and only aspects of those intelligences that can be measured by one-size-fits-all IQ tests and discipline-based standardized testing that measures momentary retention of discrete bits of knowledge (1983/1985, 16–18). In reality, Gardner says, people have many different intelligences that interact with one another and are configured differently in everyone, and schools, instead of using a deficit approach to education, should offer students myriad ways to succeed and multiple ways in which to learn (1995, 208). Drama incorporates more of the intelligences Gardner delineates than any other pedagogical tool. Students involved in classroom drama will use and develop their verbal-linguistic and logical skills in the course of putting their thoughts into language and presenting arguments or making a point. They develop bodily-kinesthetic abilities through having opportunities to use their whole bodies in a learning experience, exploring the ways bodies move in space and time. Many drama activities also incorporate the arts of music, drawing, sculpture, and film, giving students with strengths in these areas opportunities to demonstrate their abilities and develop them further. Drama also helps students develop their intrapersonal intelligence as they draw upon their own feelings and experiences and reflect on what they have learned about themselves through the course of a drama.

All drama work also draws heavily on interpersonal intelligence, as students interact with, respond to, and cooperate with one another to accomplish their goals. Drama work is social. It places the student in a context in which he must work with others, in which people must try on various viewpoints to communicate and make things happen. It is here that preconceived notions and prejudices are tested in a community forum where they can be challenged and refuted. It is here that people prepare themselves to test out actions in the real world, where standing up to a homophobic character in a drama, for example, may lead directly to addressing homophobia in a real-life situation.

Educational Drama

Any form of dramatic activity can be considered educational drama, from a play by Shakespeare to a simple role-play in a classroom about a conflict in a student's life, depending upon how that activity is framed. This book focuses upon a few forms of educational drama, those that can be easily facilitated by people without a drama background and can be useful in secondary classrooms across the curriculum, particularly when working with sensitive social issues that have deep emotional roots.

In this country, the primary way in which drama is brought into classrooms is through *scripted plays*, usually from the Western literary canon. Students are assigned roles and given lines to memorize or are asked to read parts out loud or stage scenes as a way to help bring difficult historical and linguistic dramatic texts to life. Readers theater (McCaslin 1990) is another way in which scripted plays are enacted in classrooms. This also has become a popular method for transforming narrative literary texts into dramatic scripts for the classroom. Each student takes a character's part and reads from a text using minimal gestures and facial expressions (263–75). To help them step into role less self-consciously, English teachers with some experience in theater will also introduce theater games to help students develop their sensory skills and concentration abilities (Spolin 1986; Cohen 1984; Chekhov 1953; etc.).

Beginning in the 1950s with the publication of Peter Slade's *Child Drama* (1954), educators with some background in the dramatic arts have developed drama strategies designed to help children express themselves and learn social skills. This is often referred to as *drama for personal development*. These strategies are most widely used in early childhood and lower elementary school classrooms. In this context, drama is seen as an extension of children's play, the primary way in which children learn. In the United States, this form of drama is best known as *creative drama* (Slade 1954; Courtney 1980; Way 1972; McCaslin 1990).

Drama across the curriculum was developed and popularized primarily by British and Irish educators Dorothy Heathcote, Gavin Bolton, Cecily O'Neill, and Jonothan Neelands and is more widespread in other English-speaking countries than in the United States. In this style of work, students become immersed in extended drama experiences while in role, usually directed by teachers in role. By stepping into several roles themselves, they explore different viewpoints of people unlike themselves. Reflection on the feelings and ideas that come up during the drama are an important part of the experience (Bolton 1992; Heathcote & Bolton 1995; Neelands 1984, 1990; O'Neill 1995; O'Neill & Lambert 1988).

Brazilian theater director, educator, and political activist Augusto Boal (1974/1985, 1992) developed his Theatre of the Oppressed as a tool for political organizing in the 1960s. Because Boal is the most well-known proponent of this *socially critical drama practice,* many people worldwide have studied with him and many educators have adapted some of his strategies for their own classrooms. Others, such as Australian drama educator Edward Errington, have developed their own socially critical drama practices. These practices, unlike drama for personal development or drama across the curriculum, do not depend on teachers working in role, directing and leading students to insights. These practices have more of a social and political focus, similar to Theatre of the Oppressed.

The theatre-in-education (TIE) movement, while drawing upon many drama-in-education strategies, relies heavily upon Boal's Theatre of the Oppressed (Jackson 1993). Professional actors, or sometimes peer educators, present dramatic situations and work with young audiences to reflect on the complexities of the personal, social, and political dynamics of the presentation and how it relates to the students' everyday worlds. Groups such as the Creative Arts Team at NYU are often invited into classrooms and schools to help students cope with social issues such as HIV/AIDS, violence, sexual abuse, and drugs (Boal 1974/1985, 1992; Errington 1992; Jackson 1993).

If I had to label my drama practice, I would call it *queer, feminist, multicultural, and social activist.* My approach includes all of the aforementioned drama strategies and ideas, but in the context of creating a supportive yet challenging democratic learning environment. In such an environment, student voices are valued and power is shared, differences are acknowledged and valued along with shared experiences, and emotions are valued along with intellect. The curriculum brings marginalized and previously suppressed voices to the center of inquiry, including those shaped by gender and sexuality, along with those shaped by race, ethnicity, social class, and ability, for the purpose of changing consciousness and taking action to create a more just and equitable society. Autobiography and consciousness raising are important features of this work, and process is always emphasized, even when a formal presentation is involved (Fisher 1987; Schutzman & Cohen-Cruz 1994; Weiler 1991).

For all these reasons, people who participate in multidimensional educational drama workshops tend to delve deeply into the work and broaden their learning experience. Many people walk away feeling transformed, others with a compelling question they wish to pursue or a new way of perceiving themselves and others. Many participants describe themselves as more empowered to address questions of difference in their daily and professional lives.

About the Dramas in This Book

The book contains descriptions of several types of drama workshops I have developed and conducted in educational settings. These workshops, devised primarily in the early and mid-1990s, address only a few issues related to sexual orientation, although the role-play in Chapter 1, based upon Peter Noel and Robert Marriott's article (1993), specifically includes a transgender character. I also include several resources relating to the effects of transphobia on youth in the bibliography that can be incorporated into a few of the workshops in the book, and which I hope to incorporate into future workshops that address transgender, transsexual, intersexual, and bisexual issues more extensively.

Addressing bisexuality and trans identity in work around sexual orientation and gender diversity is critical. Bisexuality is still not well understood in lesbian and gay communities, and certainly not in the heterosexual world, with dire consequences for people at risk for contracting sexually transmitted diseases. And trans youth, particularly young people of color and all who visibly transgress normative gender roles, are at great risk for being suspended or expelled from school, becoming homeless, and being subjected to emotional and physical violence.

The first chapter contains three role-plays. One is about a queer-bashing experience; the second is about how a school tackles related issues of racism and homophobia; and the third is a community meeting in which community members discuss pervasive homophobia and get to know the community's gay, lesbian, bisexual, and trans members whose existence is often ignored.

The purpose of the first role-play is to help students explore different points of view and the causes for homophobic violence. In the second role-play a fictional school community examines links between racism and homophobia and how to make the environment safer and more supportive for everyone. In the third role-play, students play the roles of people in a community in order to see what they can do collectively to lessen homophobia.

Chapter 2 introduces the topic of lesbian- and gay-headed families as well as how homophobia hurts everyone. It also raises the question of the role of emotionally charged discourse in classrooms and the question of teachers sharing personal experiences with students. The chapter includes an essay about working with a short one-act play about a lesbian mother and her son, who has difficulty accepting his mother's sexual identity. It talks about working with the script in two settings: a high school classroom and a teacher education classroom. The chapter also contains the script of the play, *garbage can blues*.

Chapter 3 contains three multifaceted drama experiences that have several different components and themes but a common structure. The first workshop explores the theme of lesbian and gay marriage; the second explores heterosexism through the lens of the high school prom; and the third examines the intersections between homophobic and racial violence, building on the simple role-play in Chapter 1.

In each workshop a facilitator guides participants through an improvised scenario, giving them direct instructions when necessary, narrating within a story, and periodically stepping into role himself to deepen the dramatic action. Although tightly guided by the leader within the framework of a story line, many activities in the workshops are designed to be self-directed by the participants. At critical moments the facilitator does what British drama specialist Gavin Bolton (1992a) calls "pushing the button"—the leader relinquishes control to empower participants to solve a problem themselves.

The workshops are all designed to accomplish several goals. In each drama, participants are given opportunities to play several different roles in order to examine sexual orientation from various viewpoints. They are asked to call upon and use what they know while simultaneously being introduced to new knowledge. They are given a chance to incorporate that knowledge into their experience in role. They are also asked to make meaning of the drama experience through discussion, writing, drawing, constructing objects, creating songs or *tableaux vivants,* or choreographing movement. Finally, each workshop includes time for reflection—ideally, participants can both reflect on what has happened through writing and discuss with the group what they have learned and what questions remain.

Chapter 4 takes a socially critical drama approach. These dramas decenter the teacher and the students take primary control of the activity. The chapter gives examples of using a variation on Augusto Boal's Forum Theatre techniques (1992), in which one group of students frame a problem and enact the problem to a point of tension. They then invite other students to try different approaches to reach a resolution. One forum focuses exclusively on what is meant by lesbian identity. In the other two, teachers, administrators, guidance counselors, lesbian and gay students, and their parents struggle with being in the closet about queer identity, ways to support sexual minority youth in schools, and how to overcome obstacles presented by homophobia.

I give fairly precise directions for and descriptions of each workshop presented in this book. However, teachers should feel free to interpret and revise these workshops to suit their own needs. For example, one person may not want to use the same scenarios in Chapter 1 but may want to keep the basic idea of a community forum. Another person may not want to enact *garbage can blues* but may use another short script or have her students develop their own scripts. Teachers may also want to investigate different topics in their own multifaceted dramas based upon their students' current interests and concerns. In any of these dramas, teachers may introduce different characters and different conflicts.

Drama Structures

I begin with workshops that have a simple structure and move to progressively more complex scenarios. Each drama activity that is described incorporates the introduction of new knowledge as well as drama learning goals to help participants incorporate what they are learning into what they already know. (I have included materials in the appendix that I have received permission to reprint to facilitate and enhance the dramas. I often find myself drawing upon daily and weekly newspaper articles to shape or supplement a drama. Because of prohibitive costs, I was not able to reprint most of the articles I have drawn upon in my own workshops in this book, although I have included references that will help educators locate ones that interest them.) Each activity is designed to help people better understand sexual orientation and gender diversity. In addition to understanding, the workshops also emphasize the importance of taking action to create safer and more welcoming schools for all students, including students who do not fit into traditional sexual and gender norms.

The workshops are designed for use across the curriculum. They can be easily adapted for English, social studies, health, art, music, dance, physical education, and theater classes, as well as guidance groups. Some of the drama experiences depend upon a facilitator who is willing to step in and out of role, perhaps with the assistance of a costume piece or prop. However, team-led workshops are very exciting and provide excellent collaborative interdisciplinary opportunities for teachers and students to work together.

For teachers who have never used drama as a teaching strategy before, this book provides all the necessary guidance needed to get started and to succeed. However, it is true that drama is unpredictable. We can never know what will happen when someone steps into role and interacts with someone else in role, but we can get an idea from what has occurred in similar situations. Therefore, I have provided examples of how participants have responded to these workshops as a way to help teachers become more confident in their ability to meet unknown challenges.

These dramas also do not require participants to have background knowledge in LGBT issues. Prior to a workshop, facilitators and classroom teachers might want to disseminate materials that give participants some exposure to the content area that the workshop will address. Such materials can also be introduced during the workshops or distributed at the end to help participants do further research on questions that emerge during the workshop.

It is up to the facilitator to help create an atmosphere of trust and security by helping people get to know one another and by introducing basic guidelines that are required for classroom interaction. People also need to know up front what will be expected of them, that someone will always be there to guide them through activities that they may not find easy, and that everything that happens in the drama will depend upon their cooperation and input.

One of the major difficulties potential participants have with drama work is that they initially equate drama with theater and memorizing scripts; they get nervous that they will be expected to perform as actors in front of an audience. Emphasizing some of the following distinctions between drama-in-education and theater for performance will help ease tensions. For example, in a drama workshop, people are not divided into the categories of performers and audience members. Everyone is audience for everyone else; everyone is a participant. There is nothing to memorize, just an opportunity to engage in an experience and cooperate and collaborate with others to reach new understandings. Nothing someone says or does in a drama is wrong. People are encouraged to express their honest feelings and ideas in order to be able to examine them in a nonjudgmental way in the course of a drama experience and by reflecting upon them afterward.

But there are also factors that drama workshops do have in common with theater. For example, both actors and drama participants do step into roles. In drama, however, people step into role for the purpose of becoming immersed in experience and then being able to reflect on that experience. One does not engage in drama-in-education for the sake of performance or entertainment. Costumes and props used in theater also are useful in drama work, particularly as a way to facilitate role-playing, achieve emotional distance, or to simply distinguish among multiple roles. For theater to work, the audience as well as the actors need to agree to a willing suspension of disbelief. In other words, everyone knows that what is happening on stage, at the moment, is a fiction, or at best a consciously constructed moment of reality in which everyone is in control. Participants in a drama must also be willing to suspend disbelief. The difference rests in purpose. Although aesthetics also are involved in drama, and may heighten engagement and enhance learning, the purpose of the drama experience is to help us better analyze the issues and topics we are exploring, which is particularly important when they have a strong emotional component.

Although it is not possible to prepare people psychologically for everything that will happen in the course of a drama, introductory comments by the workshop leader about the differences and similarities between drama and theater and what participants might expect to happen in general puts people at ease. It lets them know that what they will be asked to do is much different and much less threatening than they had feared. It is also important to let people know that they will not be forced to do anything they do not want to do. It is perfectly fine for participants in a drama to excuse themselves from portions of the drama and then come back in at a later time, as long as they do not interfere with the participation of others.

Warm-Ups

Facilitators may choose to start one of these workshops with a warm-up activity. The purpose of such action is to help people make the transition from a purely intellectual classroom experience to one that involves mind, body, and emotions, and, if they are not acquainted, to assist them in getting to know one another. Warm-up activities work best when they are related to the content of the workshop and help the participants step more easily into role.

Some people find separate warm-up activities useful. For example, participants in a workshop may be asked to move around the room, noticing everything in the environment. Eventually they are asked to notice one another and occasionally make eye contact and break eye contact. Soon after, they may be asked to step into role as teachers getting ready for work in the morning, students getting ready for school, or parents getting ready to leave the house. They may choose a name, determine how they like to dress, and visualize something they like to do, what they like to read, what kind of music they like to listen to. They then begin to get ready, going through all the steps of their morning ritual. They start out slowly and eventually have to rush to get ready. The warm-up ends when the participants gather together in the place they are going to, greet their peers and colleagues at work or school, and take a seat.

Another warm-up activity I have used involves people changing gender roles. Participants find their own space in which to stand or sit. They then mime an everyday activity, something simple and repetitive they can continue doing without tiring easily. It should be something they might do at home or work, when on vacation, and so on. They keep doing the motion and eventually say the first word or phrase that comes to mind, whether it seems related to the motion or not.

Once they become comfortable, they are asked to begin another activity or transform the one they are doing as if they saw themselves in another gender position in society. It is important to remind participants not to worry about looking silly and to remind them that everyone is doing the same thing, concentrating on herself and not others. It is important to emphasize that there is no right or wrong. When they have done the movement and sound work for a while, participants discuss how the activity they did changed when they switched genders and how they felt stepping into another gender role.

I have also had students warm up by reading homoerotic poems by authors such as Emily Dickinson, Langston Hughes, and Walt Whitman, poets who addressed lesbian and gay themes in their work. These readings often lead to very interesting and eye-opening discussions about sexual identity and censorship.

Other activities I have found effective are activities like "Diversity Balloons" from *Homophobia: How We All Pay the Price* (Blumenfeld 1992, 284). This multipurpose exercise immediately gets participants working together as a community in a lighthearted way while introducing them to language and concepts that may be unfamiliar or uncomfortable. It is designed to break the ice and get people moving around, something they're not used to doing in classrooms. It also helps people become familiar with language used in queer communities and the language of identity that may be unfamiliar to them, language that is rarely used in schools. Many teachers I've worked with have said they don't talk about diversity issues, particularly lesbian and gay issues, because they are afraid of using the wrong words and offending people.

Augusto Boal, in his book *Games for Actors and Non-Actors* (1992), also presents a variety of activities that could be useful in these workshops. I have used many of them, including "West Side Story" (93), in which body movement and nonverbal expression helps people understand the power of sound and movement and its influence on others.

Standard acting books are also full of exercises that might be adapted for warm-up exercises for queer-related workshops. For example, I often use "contentless scenes," scenes that are not about anything in particular, but ask students to give the scenes a queer subtext. Or we do a series of quick improvisation activities to get warmed up, with two people doing something and beginning a dialogue and then someone freezing the action, replacing one person, and beginning a new dialogue and action. Exercises such as these can be found in books such as Spolin's *Improvisations for the Theater* (1963/1983); Cohen's *Acting Power* (1978); Meisner's *On Acting* (1987); and Chekhov's *To the Actor* (1953).

However, the workshop itself may be the ideal environment for warming up participants and preparing them to take personal risks. Workshop activities build upon one another, starting with simple activities and leading to more complex interactions and conflicts. Finally, at the end of the workshop it is important to leave time for reflecting on the context and process of the workshop. Even where resolution of a problem encountered may not be possible and may not be desirable, it is important for participants to reach some closure. Such closure gives participants a chance to comfortably come out of role and be in the present moment instead of the fiction. It gives them time just to be with themselves and then to share the feelings they experienced with others.

Passionate and Satisfying Learning

Often I have heard teachers complain that trying to talk about lesbian and gay issues in their classes has been like pulling teeth. Even when they assign a gay text, their students are very reluctant to talk or write about what they've read. Drama, however, has the ability to liberate people, particularly those who resist examining beliefs that are based on social taboos and prejudices. One of drama's greatest assets is that it provokes the expression of a range of emotions in a relatively safe environment. It makes people laugh and cry, feel and think. Classes in which we work through drama to explore sexuality and gender issues may also be among our students' most remembered and well-liked learning experiences. Such work does not focus exclusively on intellectual knowledge but incorporates the emotions, the body, interpersonal communication, and intrapersonal reflection. Drama is satisfying because it encompasses the whole person. Even a teacher or student who first is resistant and mistrustful benefits, sometimes stepping into role with the concentrated focus of a professional actor and becoming the most invested participant in the story. There is no limit to what people can learn when the educational experience is emotionally satisfying and intellectually stimulating. Learning about sexual orientation and gender diversity through drama is transformative because it is both academically challenging and personally rewarding.

1

Role-Plays

Antihomophobia educators often use role-plays in sensitivity training work: bringing the lesbian or gay lover home for dinner, learning your best friend is a lesbian, coming out as gay at work, and so on (Blumenfeld 1992, 294–302). The workshops in this chapter are also simple role-plays designed to examine sexual orientation and gender identity from multiple points of view and from a broad community perspective. These role-plays are guided by a facilitator in role as a talk show host or community leader. Participants are not required to take big risks dramatically; they are not even asked to leave their seats. People just adopt a particular role and develop that character by interacting with others in a community forum while trying to resolve a problem.

This experiential approach to problem solving can be adapted to investigate complicated issues in various contexts. The exploration can take place through the stimulus of a novel, story, article, poem, or film, or the class can delve into an issue exclusive of an outside source of stimulation. The first role-play in the chapter does not require outside reading. The second is based upon an article from the *New York Times,* which the facilitator can summarize. The rights to reprint the piece were too expensive to include it here. The third role-play is designed to be used alongside an article from the *Village Voice,* which the author, Peter Noel, gave me permission to include.

Talk Show Takes on Gay/Trans Bashing*

Suggested Readings

Homophobia: How We All Pay the Price, by Warren Blumenfeld

Homophobia: A Weapon of Sexism, by Suzanne Pharr

Article from a newspaper, such as Jonathan Rabinovitz's *New York Times* article, "A School Is Split Over Boys in Skirts"

Invisible Lives: The Erasure of Transsexual and Transgendered People, by Viviane K. Namaste

Transgender Warriors, by Leslie Feinberg

The Internet also provides many resources one could use to bring home the seriousness of homophobia and transphobia in a role-play. For example, Gwendolyn Ann Smith created a website titled *Remembering Our Dead,* which, she explains, is "dedicated to preserving the memory of individuals murdered by transgender hate and killed by transgender prejudice." The site, *<www.gender.org/remember>,* lists the names of approximately two hundred trans people who have been murdered.

Materials

Role cards

To prepare for this role-play, students are first are asked to read an article that examines homophobia or transphobia, for example, the introduction to Warren Blumenfeld's book *Homophobia: How We All Pay the Price* (1992), a chapter from Suzanne Pharr's *Homophobia: A Weapon of Sexism* (1988), a chapter from Vivane K. Namaste's *Invisible Lives: The Erasure of Transsexual and Transgendered People* (2000), or Leslie Feinberg's *Transgender Warriors* (1997), and to respond in writing. Such responses prepare students to engage in a role-play by first asking them to articulate their present beliefs and ideas. One student doing this assignment wrote:

> Although I think everyone has a right to their own beliefs, and that nobody has a right to distinguish what is "proper" and "improper" for someone else, I still find myself being prejudiced. I think to myself: "If my child ever was 'that' then what would I do?"

---

* This role-play was initially developed by Becca Chase and myself for a first-year composition class she taught in 1993. Dr. Chase currently teaches English Education at Illinois State University.

The next day in class, students are asked to choose a role to play related to an incident in which a lesbian, trans, gay, or bisexual person is bashed. They will choose a role from a group of already marked and prefolded role cards (cut up, used file folders suit the purpose well) labeled with the following roles: victim, perpetrator, victim's lover, perpetrator's lover, perpetrator's friend, victim's family member(s), victim's coworker, social worker or psychotherapist, police officer, and religious leader. After choosing the roles they will play, they add their own names or names they have made up for the purpose, place the cards on their desks for everyone to see, and take seats in a circle. (Having students choose their own roles is preferable. In this way students more easily buy into the fictional situation they are creating. But students can also be asked to pull a role card from a hat or switch with another student to take a role they feel more ready to enact.)

Once everyone is seated, to begin the role-play, the facilitator in role as a TV talk show host comments upon how difficult it was to get everyone who was involved in the queer-bashing incident to sit down together in front of a live TV audience. The host asks the victim to begin speaking by discussing what happened during the incident and then calls on someone else to respond, perhaps the basher. The host assists the go-around by directing questions to each participant, calling on those who were most closely affected by the incident first, inviting others to speak later, and seeking perspectives from the people in role as professionals, who can be especially useful in cooling down a heated exchange. This go-around continues until everyone with a role card has spoken at least once. In one such discussion, a student in role as the father of a lesbian who had been beaten exclaimed:

> She has failed me, shamed me in front of my friends and family. What do you think it's like for me to go to work? I don't like getting flak from the guys, I tell you. I don't know what went wrong. It's not my fault, it's her mother's.

Later, her sister dropped her own bombshell: "I understand what it's like to be ostracized," she said, "because I'm bisexual."

At this point, the father slapped his forehead in disbelief, jumped out of his chair, and stormed out of the room. Everyone in the room froze in stunned silence. But in the next moment the drama continued. The students were so totally involved that the outburst was accepted as part of the drama.

After the role-play, students write about what it was like to step into their roles and share their experience with others in the class. For example, people often react with nervous, edgy laughter when they are uncomfortable about a situation like this, and it is important to discuss this phenomenon when it arises. One student was upset by what seemed like inappropriate laughter.

Several people kept bursting into laughter when people said very homophobic things. I understand that the ideas expressed were those of the characters and not necessarily those of the students, but it still hurt somewhat just to hear those hateful words and it made me wonder when I heard those aforementioned people laugh. Just what is it they find so amusing about this hatred?

Another student commented on the usefulness of role-playing about homophobia:

I think there are a lot more people out there that think homosexuality is wrong than are noticeable. [Often] you'll have people in a classroom arguing the politically correct point of view. That comes from homosexuality still not being a comfortable classroom discussion topic. At least with role-playing you get to hear all the sides without having people ostracized for their views.

In the go-around, the participants are asked to listen for any differences between the responses of those who stepped into role as victim and perpetrator and those close to them, between LGBT people and heterosexuals, and between those who were directly and peripherally involved. They are also asked to think about anything they have seen in the media about people who have been involved in homophobic or transphobic attacks as victims or perpetrators and compare real incidents to what the role-play created. They are asked to look at what was similar and different, where stereotypes came into play, and what suggestions they have for making the role-play more realistic. Finally, students are asked to reflect on what can be done to decrease homophobic and transphobic attitudes and violence in the real world, based upon the characters they created in the role-play.

It Can Happen Here: Homophobia and Racism at Pleasantville High

Suggested Readings

Article from a newspaper, such as Evelyn Nieves' *New York Times* article, "Attacks on a Gay Teen-Ager Prompt Outrage and Soul-Searching"

"Youth Bring Gay Rights Movement to School," Lambda Legal Defense and Education Fund (see appendix)

PFLAG fact sheet (see appendix)

Materials

Gay/Straight Alliance flier (see appendix)

Writing in role handout (see p. 23)

Role cards

Using a text or a description of an event to shape their drama, participants in this role-play investigate ways in which a school community can respond to racist and homophobic violence. To prepare for the role-play, students read or the facilitator summarizes an article from the *New York Times* (Nieves 1999) about a student in California who was brutally beaten and had the letters *FAG* scratched into his stomach and arms. This occurred shortly after he came out and announced the formation of a gay/straight alliance at his high school. The article also describes this community's history of racism toward African American and Asian American people and draws links between homophobic and racist violence. People in this role-play step into roles as people in the high school and general community of a nearby California town.

The facilitator steps into role as the principal and asks community residents, whom she has invited to a meeting, to help her understand what has occurred in the nearby school, to assess whether this school community is facing similar problems, and to decide, as a community, what can be done to create a safer and more supportive environment for everyone in the community.

The principal (facilitator) will summarize or ask everyone to read the *New York Times* article to familiarize themselves with what occurred, mentioning that some people may have read about these incidents in the local papers but may not be aware that the *New York Times* picked up the story. She will also mention legal actions taken by Lambda Legal Defense and Education Fund to protect youth in schools, emphasizing the suit brought by a gay student named Jamie Nabozny, in Wisconsin, who successfully sued his school district for almost $1 million for not protecting him from homophobic violence (see appendix). She then shows the group a Gay/Straight Alliance flier (see appendix) that has been posted at Pleasantville High.

The principal should ask the participants to discuss what the *Times* article describes, including how the gay student had been taunted and jeered in the hallways and in the parking lot before this incident occurred. Someone even wrote an epithet with lighter fluid in his family's driveway. The group should also discuss the racial incidents mentioned in the article, in which white students chanted racial epithets at a football game and wore Afro wigs and face paint to mock black people. It points out that four African American parents were suing the school district. After the incident, swastikas and other hate graffiti began appearing on the high school's walls and students also performed a racially insensitive skit at the talent show. There had been other incidents throughout the years. For example, in 1995 an Asian American senior was beaten by a group of teens who shouted racial epithets and told him to go back to China, and in 1996 a white man stabbed an Asian man for no other reason than because he was Asian.

To stimulate the discussion, the principal could ask how everyone feels about the article. For example, she might ask if they see similar problems in this school, and if people feel that only a few troublemakers are causing all the problems, as the *Times* article suggests, or if there are deeper problems the community must address. It is also important to discuss whether the participants, in role, agree that the racism and homophobia described in the article are indeed linked.

The principal then asks everyone to choose a role card on which a variety of generic roles are written: parent, student, LGBT student, teacher, queer teacher, guidance counselor, religious leader, community leader, politician, businessperson, law enforcement officer, and so on, depending upon the number of participants in the group. Participants sit in a circle and write their names for everyone to see on the role card they have chosen. They are then given a handout that asks them to write in role as the character they have chosen in response to one of several questions (see p. 23 for list of questions).

The principal then asks the community members to air their concerns in a go-around, asking for a volunteer to start by reading or paraphrasing what he or she has written. From time to time, the facilitator, in role as principal, will ask people to clarify what they mean. The facilitator also may want to ask participants in role to speak to one or more of the issues they have raised in some depth and to try to come up with some practical solutions to the problems they are posing.

Reflecting on the role-play afterward, participants should be asked to speak about what it was like stepping into role and writing in role, what they learned about the concerns of communities such as this and the issues involved, and what they might have learned about themselves.

At one presentation of this workshop, the participants enthusiastically jumped into role immediately. The participant in role as a math teacher said that she did not have time for one more concern in her classroom. She had to get students ready for the tests. She had attendance forms to fill out and other paperwork. She just felt overwhelmed by her responsibilities and didn't want to take on one more thing.

The parent responded that it wasn't the teacher's job to educate children about homosexuality. "Parents should guide children about moral issues."

But another teacher argued that it is the school's responsibility to educate against prejudice in a democratic society. This teacher was struggling with how to introduce literature with gay themes in his classroom without provoking homophobic male students in his class to act out.

The heterosexual student said he was afraid to support gay students. "I hear a lot of stuff going on in the hallways, and I'm afraid to stick my neck out, especially since the school isn't doing anything about it. Teachers don't stop stuff from happening and make sexist and racist remarks themselves."

By the time the conversation was over, everyone was starting to work together to try to address what the school needed to do to counteract the racism and homophobia that had been reported, including the parent and the math teacher. They talked about forming a gay/straight alliance for students and teachers and educating parents, and they even challenged the principal to take a stand as a strong leader in the school and community to speak out more against prejudice of all forms. Everyone felt as if we had just gotten started by the time we had to stop.

This role-play has a variety of content and drama goals that are interrelated. The *New York Times* article and information about the Jamie Nabozny lawsuit give the participants important information to incorporate into any follow-up assignments or research projects about the particular types of violence directed against lesbians, gays, bisexuals, and trans people; the ways in which racism and homophobia are often linked; and what actions people have taken to address these grievances. The packet given to participants to peruse during the role-play should also contain a summary of typical ways in which LGBT students are treated in schools and the effects of these behaviors, prepared by groups such as Parents, Families, and Friends of Lesbians and Gays (PFLAG); the Education Coalition on Lesbian and Gay Youth (ECOLaGY); the Gay, Lesbian, and Straight Education Network (GLSEN); the Hetrick-Martin Institute; and others, which they can incorporate into their work.

Giving people the opportunity to step into roles as members of a community affected by racism and homophobia helps them consolidate the information they have gleaned about different groups in the community. Dramatically, stepping into role as people who are directly affected by homophobia and racism is an important part of the work, allowing people to bring their own concerns and experiences to the foreground in the role of someone else. This often allows people to express feelings and ideas they would not otherwise express and to experience the way other people perceive their feelings and ideas.

Write in Role in Response to One or More of the Following Questions

1. What problems do you face in relation to racism and/or homophobia as a person in your role? What concerns do you have about these issues?

2. What is the relationship between the racist and homophobic violence we are seeing in this community? Do you have any suggestions for coalition building?

3. What is the role of parents in the moral development of children?

4. What is the responsibility of our schools in the moral development of children and in educating against prejudice?

5. As someone concerned with hate crimes and discrimination, what arguments do you need to prepare yourself to address?

6. Does the article in the *New York Times* exaggerate the problems we have in our communities or portray them accurately? What do you think about the argument some in the community raise that it is just a small group of troublemakers who are causing all the problems?

Homophobia and Homosexuality in a Caribbean American Community

Suggested Readings

"Batty Boys in Babylon: Can Gay West Indians Survive the 'Boom Bye Bye' Posses?" by Peter Noel with Robert Marriott (see appendix pp. 93–110)

Supplementary Readings

"Jeers, Threats Greet Gays in South Boston Parade," by Don Aucion and Andy Dabilis

Other articles about homophobia in different ethnic communities may be found in local newspapers and on the Internet. On May 10, 1993, several articles appeared in the *New York Times* and the *Jerusalem Post* about Orthodox Jewish groups protesting the inclusion of gays in the Israel Day Parade.

Materials

List of characters and page numbers on which characters appear (see pp. 30–31)

Sample questions for students-in-role (see pp. 31–32)

This role-play, about homophobia and homosexuality in the Caribbean community in Brooklyn, New York, is based upon an ethnographic study published as an article in the *Village Voice*, by Peter Noel with Robert Marriott (1993). Students in the classroom step into role as people in the article to discuss homophobia in a community setting and strategize ways for the community to respond to intolerance demonstrated against sexual minorities in the community.

The structure of this drama is similar to the queer-bashing drama. But, rather than read an article for background, this time students read an article that creates the foundation for their work and the characters they will play. The article "Batty Boys in Babylon: Can Gay West Indians Survive the 'Boom Bye Bye' Posses?" vividly depicts homophobia in Brooklyn's Caribbean community. It also sympathetically portrays several Caribbean lesbians, gay men, bisexuals, and trans people.

The graphic descriptions of homophobic violence in this article, along with use of profanity and sexual language, may prevent its widespread use in high schools. In the venue in which I used it there were no problems, but many high school teachers may find it more difficult to introduce in their classrooms. In that case, the article could be excerpted.

Much of the article features dialogue in a variety of Caribbean dialects, and some students may find the reading challenging. But this is an important aspect of its literary and cultural value. Working with this article is an excellent way to help students learn to appreciate multiple and diverse literacies as well as affirm the possible variety of literacies of students in the class.

Despite the article's challenges, I have included it in the appendix and developed the role-play to be used alongside it. The article's poignancy, enhanced by its rich attention to details, and the realistic intensity of the language enable it to convey to young people that homophobia is a serious problem they cannot ignore. The article is one of the most effective stimuli I have used to facilitate deep discussion and cross-cultural understanding about hatred toward and fear of sexual and gender minorities.

In addition to reading the Noel and Marriott piece, I also require students to read articles about homophobia in other communities to counter any possibility of racist stereotyping and to reinforce that homophobia is not exclusive to the Caribbean community. For example, we read articles about the Irish Lesbian and Gay Organization trying to march in the St. Patrick's Day Parade and about Jewish lesbians and gays trying to march in the Israel Day Parade.

This role-play requires a little more preparation than the previous ones. Students need to do a careful reading of a difficult text and become familiar with the characters that are discussed. A sheet listing the characters in the article, short descriptions of each, and page numbers where they can be found helps students become familiar with their character more easily and allows them to go back quickly through the text to reread sections that will help them better understand the parts they will each play. Students will also have the experience of discussing manifestations of homophobia in other communities before tackling the Noel and Marriott piece in depth. If time allows, in addition to reading newspaper articles, a class session can be set aside for a guest speaker who is actively and publicly combating homophobia. If possible, it would be good to invite a representative from an ethnically identified gay organization, such as the Irish Lesbian and Gay Organization in New York (ILGO). If no such representative is available, a member of Parents, Families, and Friends of Lesbians and Gays; the Gay, Lesbian, and Straight Education Network; or another national or local organization would also be beneficial. Inviting such activists not only reinforces the fact that homophobia is pervasive but also demonstrates that people have been fighting back.

Like the other role-plays in this book, the teacher is in role, but this time as a guest invited by community leaders to facilitate a community discussion about the article and its possible repercussions. This guest calls on people from the community to speak and facilitates discussion. I have included a list of questions I used as the facilitator to stimulate the discussion and involve everyone in the discussion (see pp. 31–32). The students in the class assume roles of people from the community, community leaders, social service professionals, and interested citizens, all of whom are mentioned in the article.

The facilitator, to encourage dialogue and increase dramatic momentum, might begin the discussion with a question such as "What do you think about Peter Noel and Robert Marriott publishing such an article about our community?" and call first on someone who might have a lot to say. I chose instead to structure the first part of our discussion carefully and asked the student in role as Dr. Blake to set the tone for the community meeting. While other students wrote in role in response to questions I prepared in advance (see list of questions for students-in-role on pp. 31–32), Dr. Blake and I sat down to prepare his opening statement. Spending the time thinking about their characters and how they might respond to the facilitator's questions in advance helped the students get more comfortable and ready to participate more actively in the role-play.

After the initial round of questions, the discussion could go in many different directions. Although the facilitator may want to focus the discussion on particular issues at a particular time, it is important to give the students as much autonomy and control as possible over the direction the discussion takes. However, the facilitator is in a position to make sure that arguments do not get out of hand and that everyone has a chance to speak. As in the other role-plays, calling on professionals in the community to calm heated debates and making sure that everyone's voice is heard are the primary tasks of the facilitator.

The Noel and Marriott article does not focus on the ways in which many people in the Caribbean community also accept and support sexual minorities, although some characters in the article are supportive. In the role-play, the facilitator tries to encourage more active community support for its lesbian, gay, bisexual, and trans members. One of educational drama's special features is its ability to help make a difficult situation less hopeless by giving more of a voice to people who wish to change negative views and behaviors.

The purpose of this role-play is to open up the discussion further about homosexuality and to offer a context in which all feelings about the issue can be aired in a safe environment. Unless negative feelings are brought to the surface, they cannot be examined. Often students can say things in the role of someone else that they are not otherwise comfortable voicing because they are afraid of being judged.

The objective of the initial portion of the drama is to air all points of view in the community as these voices are represented in the article and as students embellish upon them. It is also possible that in the course of the drama, some of the characters may be persuaded to change their minds. In introductory remarks, the facilitator should point out that characters may change their position as a result of the discussion and that students may change the characters slightly if they feel they cannot play the characters exactly as written, for one reason or another. However, it is important to the learning process that students be able to articulate why a character changed in a later reflection on the activity.

Before the role-play, students are asked to write in role about how their own character relates to the topic of homosexuality and violence against gays. After the role-play, students are asked to write in role about the character they played, summarizing what they said during the role-play and adding anything they did not have a chance to say during the drama. Everyone then shares their writing aloud, which adds yet another layer of meaning. In one class, some students stepped out of role for this reflective writing. The student who played Slicksta, a Jamaican man who bashed gay men, was disturbed because it didn't seem to him that other people in the class were willing to take the same risks he did to make his character believable. He was particularly upset with the student who played Buju Banton because that student did not express as much hostility toward gays as he did and as the article indicated Buju Banton felt. The student who played Slicksta was not aware that the student who played Buju Banton was bisexual and had difficulty, understandably, distancing himself enough to play the role believably.

Another student said she also had difficulty playing the role of someone who was homophobic. She wrote:

> I must say it was really hard for me to act as Desmond's stepfather because he's so anti-gay and I'm not. It was difficult to say things in that character. I felt like crying because I so deeply believe that everyone has a right to live however they want. Some people were better in their roles than me. I guess I let my emotions interfere too much. I should learn that in some situations they aren't needed but with this topic I found it particularly hard not to be emotional.

As moderator, I think it is important to help students make a commitment to the roles they are playing and stay focused on their characters. But it is also important to point out that it is difficult emotionally to play a role that is either very different from ourselves or very close to ourselves, and that we have to take care of ourselves and each other in this work. That is why it is important not to judge ourselves or anyone else but to just note what we are feeling while in role.

Despite the difficulties some students found in stepping into roles, their role work seemed to deepen their understanding of the issues. As one student wrote:

> Playing a role of a particular character, I think, helped each of my class-mates and me to know and understand more about the certain character's pain, anguish, frustration and thinking. Although there were many hostile remarks and hatred in the conversation I believe that the discussion is the first important step towards resolving differences.

Other students did write in role. In one class, the character of Slicksta made a strong impression on everyone when he read out loud:

> All this ballyhoo about "batty bwoys." It's nothing but ballyhoo man. God never created man to love another man or a woman to love another woman. They break the rules, they pay, man.

He played his role so intensely and believably that many students reacted to his characterization by trying to figure out how a community can deal with attitudes such as his. The heterosexually identified Caribbean student in role as Colin Robinson, a leader in the Caribbean gay community, movingly responded:

> I think we still have a long way to go. Figures like Slicksta represent a large population of people in West Indian society who cannot accept any homo-sexuality. But it was positive to have such a meeting, because now we are out in the open. Also, people can see that Slicksta made a mockery of him-self at the meeting. People seemed to view his way of thinking as childish, immature, and even humorous. I think this is an important first step to an integrated society.

Another student, writing as Desmond's stepfather, emphasized how im-portant honesty was and while in role encouraged his stepson to come out to his mother. He said that this was the first step toward resolving problems.

The student who played Lopinot, a Trinidadian, talked about how diffi-cult it was to be out in his community and experience the hostility of others. But he too talked about the community meeting in a positive way:

> I'm happy now since more people like me were here today at the meeting than there were of people like Slicksta. I even met a cute guy named Desmond who also was looking for a friend.

The drama work also inspired tremendous honesty. It gave students permission to share and examine their own prejudices, without fearing judgment. For example, in reflecting on the drama experience, one student wrote:

> My parents do not really say anything about sex at home or to me. I pretty much learn about sex through books and people. I found out that homosexuals were viewed as abnormal, so I tried to stay away from them. I grew up in a society that was anti-gay. I remember the times when I was a little kid, I would joke along with people in making fun of homosexuals. Also I would act gay to make people laugh. As I matured, I accepted homosexuals as they are, but inside of me was still homophobic.

The drama made some students wonder why the violence against gay people is so intense.

> Whenever I read or hear about these hate crimes the same question springs to mind, "why do they happen?" I've never been able to figure that one out. Sure, everyone, including me, has their own prejudices, but that's no reason to go around killing people. What if everyone thought that hatred is the perfect excuse for violence? That would definitely solve any problem of over-population. So, why isn't everyone like that? Why can one person control his prejudices while another person kills because of them?

Other students speculated about why homophobia exists and examined its relationship to other forms of prejudice within their own communities. One Chinese American student wrote:

> To my way of thinking, attacks on homosexuals are like attacks on Blacks, Asians . . . because they are different. We all know that segregation (blacks having to sit in the back of the bus sort of thing) is wrong. We all know that racial remarks and attacks are wrong but I don't understand our tolerance of attacks on homosexuals because of their sexual preference. We all look back at the fight the Jews, Chinese, Hispanics, etc. had to go through for equal rights and we praise them on their courageousness, but we don't see— we don't connect the fact that the homosexuals are fighting for those same rights.

Discussion and writing that develop through immersion in a drama experience are rich in detail, problematizing, and reflection, some of the writing areas that are most troublesome for high school students and young writers in general. Initially, a white female student in my class complained about how hard the Noel and Marriott article was to understand because of its use of dialect. She complained that the text was "undecipherable" for her. Then in class, we read portions aloud, which she said really helped her to understand it and enabled her to go back and read it again herself. As a result, she became very involved in the discussion and this helped her link what was going on in her own life to the article. She wrote in her log:

> Halfway through the article, I found myself getting really angry. I kept thinking about the difference between me and my brother. My brother—the essential homophobe—and me—miss bleeding-heart liberal; acceptor-of-all. Why are we so different? Why do we think so differently when we're only three years apart? Was it the way we were brought up or the experiences we had that made us different?

She also commented on the importance of having had the experience of reading a text in an unfamiliar dialect and learning how to appreciate it.

The most moving part of the role-play was the male student who voluntarily stepped into the role of Zanelia, Peter Noel's eleven-year-old daughter. Although her appearance in the article was brief, he developed her character by poignantly reflecting on her deep conflict between her love for her uncle and her love for the music that called for his death. This was the first time I saw this student engage in a meaningful way in anything we read that semester.

Simple role-plays such as these, in which everyone plays a role, and which do not even require students to leave their seats, get everyone involved in the learning process. They expose students to multiple points of view and can help them think more clearly about subjects they have only explored superficially. Such role-plays, because of the interest they stimulate, can also lead to further reading, as well as writing that is more thoughtful and has more voice and emotional depth.

Roles from "Batty Boys in Babylon"
(Page numbers refer to the article in the appendix, pp. 93–110. This list includes only characters mentioned in this chapter.)

1. Dr. Luther Blake—Jamaican-born political and educational consultant. p. 110
2. Buju Banton—West Indian dancehall singer. pp. 94, 96, 100, 107–09
3. Moi Renee—Gay transgender Jamaican performance artist. pp. 98–99, 102
4. Naphthali—Moi Renee's brother, and a member of the Twelve Tribes of Israel, an offshoot of the Rastafari movement. p. 102
5. Winsome—Jamaican lesbian, a Twelve Tribes member. pp. 103–04
6. Slicksta—Jamaican man who bashes gay men. pp. 93–96
7. Dr. Marco Mason—Panamanian sociologist. p. 94

8. Yula—Rebel Rasta lesbian. pp. 103–04
9. Desmond's stepfather—Antiguan stepfather of Guyanese gay man. p. 101
10. Desmond—Guyanese gay man. pp. 101–02
11. Lopinot's mother—Mother of Trinidadian gay man. p. 102
12. Ambakaila—Trinidadian bisexual woman. pp. 104–05
13. Sally Jean—White girlfriend of Ambakaila. p. 105
14. Colin Robinson—Cochair of Gay Men of African Descent. p. 101
15. Zanelia—Peter Noel's eleven-year-old daughter. p. 107
16. Peter Noel—Trinidadian writer, author of article. pp. 106–07

Suggested Questions for Students-in-Role

Introductory Comments

1. Facilitator: Dr. Luther Blake invited me here, as someone from outside the community, to facilitate this meeting. Dr. Blake will now say something about what has brought us together tonight.

2. Dr. Blake: I have called the community together to respond to Peter Noel and Robert Marriott's article in the *Village Voice.* I think it's important that we know how people in the community feel about the article and talk about how we may want to respond to the article and the problem it discusses as a community.

Questions

3. Facilitator to Buju Banton: As a popular musician, what do you think about the way you and your music were presented in the article? Why did you refuse to talk with Mr. Noel and what do you think about your record being banned?

4. Facilitator to Moi Renee: As a victim of gay bashing and someone who has left Jamaica to live more freely as a gay man, how are you affected by Buju's lyrics?

5. Facilitator to Naphthali: You are Moi Renee's brother. What kind of relationship do you envision with him in the future? What was it like for you to read the account of how you treated your brother in the article?

6. Facilitator to Winsome: As a Twelve Triber yourself, how do you account for your attitudes toward homosexuality? Why are yours and Naphthali's attitudes so different, since he is also a member of the same sect?

7. Facilitator to Slicksta: What do you think of Dr. Blake's prediction in the article that people's attitudes will change, that they will become more tolerant? Listening to Moi Renee and Winsome today, what about them makes them sound like evil spirits to you?

8. Facilitator to Yula: What do you think about Buju and Slicksta and the way they put down zami queens (lesbians)? How does it make you feel?

9. Facilitator to Desmond's stepfather: How did your portrayal in the article make you feel? Is there something you'd like to change or add to the piece?

10. Facilitator to Desmond: Do you want to go back home? Do you think your mother will ever let you? Why or why not?

11. Facilitator to Lopinot's mother: You seem to have accepted your son for who he is. Do you have any reservations? If you have made peace with him, what would you want to say to Desmond's mother?

12. Facilitator to Ambakaila: Why didn't you go to Michael's party? What in Peter's article might help you sort out how you feel about your identity and your place in the community?

13. Facilitator to Sally Jean: Do you think it's easier for you in your community as a lesbian or bisexual than it is for Ambakaila in her community? Why?

14. Facilitator back to Ambakaila: Do you agree with Sally Jean's assessment or do you see things differently?

15. Facilitator to Colin Robinson: As a black gay man, what kind of impact do you think this article might have on the West Indian gay community? Could it make life easier or harder? Why?

16. Facilitator to Zanelia: You were having so much fun dancing to that song. How did it make you feel when your father said the song was about your uncle getting killed?

17. Facilitator to Peter Noel: What were you trying to accomplish with your article? What did you learn in the process of working on it?

18. Facilitator to Dr. Mason: Could you sum up what you heard here today? In what directions do you see us moving as a community?

Dr. Blake thanks everyone for attending the meeting and announces the next step that will be taken to address homophobia in the community.

2

Scripted Dramas

This chapter raises complex issues about conflicts that can arise in lesbian- and gay-headed families, issues that are often disregarded even in antihomophobia work. It is composed of a short play and an introductory essay that also raises important and sometimes troubling questions about the role of personal knowledge in the classroom. The tension the play depicts between a lesbian mother and her son will resonate with many parents and children who try to understand one another despite intergenerational and interpersonal barriers. At the same time, the play underscores unique concerns of particular sexual minority family members.

The scene, although fictional, is based upon real-life experiences. The conflict between mother and son is exaggerated and telescoped to let the audience experience the intensity and complexity of a difficult parent-child relationship. The relationship is further distorted through the intermediary of an inanimate object, which, from a Brechtian standpoint, also distances the characters from one another and from the audience, allowing more opportunities for reflection.

Although the characters in the play are a lesbian mother and her son, it is not necessary for the teacher who uses these materials or the actors to be lesbian, bisexual, trans, or gay; nor do the actors need formal theater experience. However, teachers who are not comfortable performing scripted material themselves could invite colleagues or students to enact the scene, yet still facilitate the intense discussion the scene may engender.

Boundaries of Classroom Discourse

Suggested Readings

Both My Mom's Names Are Judy, video produced by the Gay and Lesbian Parents Association

Free Your Mind: The Book for Gay, Lesbian and Bisexual Youth—and Their Allies, by Ellen Bass and Kate Kaufman

Homophobia: How We All Pay the Price, by Warren Blumenfeld

Jack, by A. M. Homes

Out of the Ordinary: Growing Up with Gay, Lesbian and Transgender Parents, by Noelle Howey and Ellen Samuels

From the Notebooks of Melanin Sun, by Jacqueline Woodson

"The Names on the Board: An Ohio Teacher Dares Students to Envision a New Community," by Jamie Rhein (see appendix pp. 111–12)

In 1995, I was invited into the high school classroom of one of my former inservice teacher education students to speak about my experience as a lesbian mother. She was concerned that her students never take lesbian and gay families into consideration and tend to assume that all teachers are heterosexual. We decided to stage a reading of a short one-act play I wrote about a relationship between a lesbian mother and her heterosexually identified son. I chose this piece because it also addresses how homophobia affects everyone. The classroom teacher was in role as the son and I played the mother.

The play opens with a young man, between twelve and sixteen years old, standing on stage. He thinks he hears his mother talking to him even though he sees only a garbage can. The mother sits near the garbage can, unseen by her son. In the first part of the scene the mother asks the son to do the dishes and lets him know she is not happy that he does not do his share of housework. Hearing her, and thinking it's the garbage can speaking, the young man gets more and more frustrated. A dialogue ensues in which neither mother nor son seem to be communicating with one another, except at certain key moments.

YOUNG MAN: You're not here. I just left you at home screaming about how you had too much to do, how you couldn't stand to see me laying around, listening to music when the house was such a mess. So I say a swear. And you yell, "Don't you talk to me like that, young man!" And I say, "I didn't say it to *you.*" So I decide to go out, and you say, "Don't bother to come back until you're ready to do your share around here, without me asking."

MA: If your memory is so good how come you can't remember when you're supposed to do the dishes?

YOUNG MAN: If you weren't queer, I wouldn't have any problems.

The mother keeps talking about wanting her son to take more responsibility for housework, and the son keeps blaming everything on his mother being a lesbian.

YOUNG MAN: Why can't you be like other mothers? . . . (*Very upset*) What do you think it's like for me? I can't invite my friends over. What if they find out?

MA: If you cleaned up your room you could invite your friends over.

YOUNG MAN: Everyone knows. The landlord, the whole neighborhood. You two look like a couple of guys walking down the street.

Then a turning point occurs. We overhear the mother talking on the phone with a friend, expressing empathy for her son. This gives the son the impetus to share his underlying confusion and pain with his mother.

YOUNG MAN: Ma, you there? Ma. Some kids I know beat up this guy who hangs out on the streets, said he was a fag, said he had AIDS. Ma, you hear me? (*Frustrated. Picks up garbage can and yells into it*) That's what they're going to do to me; they'll think I'm queer 'cause you're a lezzie. (*Pause*) I should have stopped them, Ma. How can I stop them? I hate myself.

MA: You wanted to stop them, that's what matters. You were only one person, what could you do? Dealing with who I am, who you are, what others think about us—it's going to get easier as you get older, I promise.

YOUNG MAN: I like this girl. But she's going out with a guy. He's older. She says she likes me better. Then this other girl who's been wanting me to ask her out—her friends told me—she asked me to go to the movies. I don't know what to do. (*Pause*) Why can't I have a beer once in a while? Sometimes I'd just like to relax in front of the TV and drink a beer. My friend with the car, we don't drink or nothing, just ride around or go to the movies.

The mother then tries to talk to her son about safe sex. Now, thoroughly embarrassed, he lashes out again.

YOUNG MAN: Jewish [change, if necessary, to indicate ethnic origin of the mother] . . . mothers aren't supposed to be garbage cans. They're supposed to look pretty, cook nice meals, keep the house clean, iron clothes, sew on buttons! [Revise to reflect the normative constructs of motherhood for the particular ethnic group.]

The scene ends by contrasting the way the son lashes out at his mother with the overly considerate behavior he demonstrates toward his father.

After the reading, an African American woman student in the high school class blurted out: "My mother is a lesbian and I hate her; I will never forgive her." Then she uttered a litany of complaints that paralleled what the young man said to his mother in the play, including that all her mother's friends look like guys and that she hates to see them walk down the streets of Harlem together because it embarrasses her. She felt tremedous conflict because her mother wanted her to like her women partners and wanted her daughter's approval. But she couldn't give it.

There were a few moments of tense silence. Struggling for words, I managed, "It must have been difficult for you to say what you said because the situation is clearly painful for you. Thank you for being so honest."

Then the teacher challenged the student by saying that she wasn't sure she was angry with her mother because she was a lesbian, but perhaps had other reasons. She also pointed out that she saw a contradiction between what the student was saying and how well the student usually understood and accepted other people's differences. Other students in the class then jumped into the conversation, pointing out how gay students at the school felt she cared about them and that one openly gay young man was always there for her when she needed someone to talk to. They asked her if she was there for him the same way. The student replied that she thought maybe I cared more about my son than her mother cared about her.

When the student reflected on the class, she remembered ways in which her mother also cared about her, but perhaps did not show her directly, similarly to the mother in the play.

A few weeks later I incorporated the play into a more extensive drama workshop I led with secondary preservice teachers in a course a colleague taught. After my colleague and I read the play this time, I mentioned the high school student's reaction to the piece. A white female student in her class responded: "My mother is a lesbian and I used to hate her too, but now I don't." She thought the high school student I described did indeed hate her mother for being a lesbian and that it was important to let her have her feelings. This student also remarked how special it was to see her own life reflected, for the first time, in this play. This led other students to talk about how they had never before considered the difficulties facing children of lesbian and gay parents and that this was something they needed to keep in mind in their own future classrooms.

When I first wrote the scene, and since then, as I worked on revisions, I had not really thought about the direct and profound impact the scene could have on an audience of young people. The high school student's vehement reaction to the piece took me by surprise. I worried that maybe it was wrong to take the play to a high school classroom because it could provoke such intense feelings in a young person. In my mind, I heard the voices of people who criticize teachers for inviting students to share strong feelings in class and for sharing strong feelings of their own with their students.

The question of teachers sharing their personal experiences in the classroom is not limited to lesbian and gay teachers. A heterosexual African American inservice high school teacher in one of my teacher education courses, when comparing her life to that of a closeted gay teacher, said that she couldn't imagine what her life would be like if she could not talk about who she was with her students. Sarah-Hope Parmeter (Parmeter & Reti 1988) makes a similar point when she speaks about gay teachers who are forced to remain in the closet. According to Parmeter, in order for our students to have the best education they can possibly have, their teachers need to "put their full energy into their teaching instead of into hiding" (57). My own pedagogical approach incorporates the use of personal narratives and sharing some of my own experience when I feel that would benefit my students.

Gisa E. Kirsch and Joy S. Ritchie, however, point out dangers in what they call "the politics of location" that reliance on personal narratives can create a new set of "master narratives" (1995, 8). This is similar to Diana Fuss' (1989) position that the sharing of personal experience "can lead to tense and harmful experiences in the classroom" because it essentializes "truth" (113).

Despite the problems that can arise when teachers share their personal narratives with their students, in certain cases the benefits seem greater than the risks. When I think about my son's experience, I know he would have had an easier time if he didn't feel he had to hide his family's differences from his peers and his teachers. If a teacher had brought an experience similar to the one I did to his classroom, or talked about all different kinds of families, or assigned an article or piece of literature to the class about lesbian- and gay-headed families, he might have been able to share his feelings, his anger toward his mother, his fears of being stigmatized. Through feedback from peers and teachers, he might have been able to see his situation in a different light or just had a chance to unlock his shame a bit.

If we had not read the play in my former student's class, I doubt that the high school student who shared her feelings would have had another chance in school to express her unhappiness in such a supportive environment. If she had not spoken up the way she had, her peers and teacher would never have had an opportunity to challenge her beliefs or point out inconsistencies in her thinking.

Preservice teachers and colleagues overwhelmed with a particular student's problems often use the excuse that they are not therapists in order to sidestep the difficult issues the student raises. I agree that classroom teachers are not trained as therapists and that our classrooms are not therapists' offices. But as teachers, in order to help our students learn, we are, in an important sense, psychologists. Any deep learning that takes place occurs on both a cognitive and an affective level as students connect what they are learning to their own lives (Dewey 1900/1990).

What takes place in the classroom can and should be enlightening, both emotionally and intellectually. This will happen more often when schools give young people a chance to talk about what has not been talked about, about what has been hidden under layers of prejudice, fear, and shame. In such environments students will also be able to bring hitherto unexamined beliefs to the surface, reflect on what occurred, and learn and be transformed by the experience. Carl Rogers (1961; 1980/1995) claims that schools can be places in which students become more fully themselves. What stands in the way, says Rogers, is that "they [American educational institutions] have focused so intently on *ideas*, have limited themselves so completely to 'education from the neck up' that the resulting narrowness is having serious social consequences" (1980/1995, 267).

Although I know that the question of boundaries in classroom discourse is not an easy one to resolve, I cannot help but think that schools and teachers can and should make more of a difference in our students' lives. Most parents do not talk with their children about tough issues; even when they want to they often feel they don't know how to. Young people do not get opportunities for constructive dialogue about gender, sexuality, and sexual identity in the home or with their peers outside school. Therefore, it is up to teachers to construct dialogues where knowledge that is suppressed or distorted in the home or on the streets can be appropriately addressed, even when these dialogues may require people to take emotional risks. If not in school, then where are our students going to learn about themselves and how to question and examine society's and their own biases?

garbage can blues*

Props and Materials

Metal garbage can and lid, plastic bag full of garbage inside

Boom box with music tape

Sound of phone ringing

Sound of car honking

Questions for classroom discussion

Nothing on stage except large, metal garbage can. Young man, between twelve and sixteen years old, dressed in latest fashion enters. He looks around, sees the garbage can, seems puzzled, takes lid off can, feels inside, sticks head in to look around, puts lid back, and walks away stage right. Ma is seated on a stool slightly upstage left from garbage can.

* First written in 1986 and revised in 1999.

MA: You haven't done the dishes yet.

YOUNG MAN: (Stops. Looks around, confused) What?

MA: I don't want to have to ask you again.

YOUNG MAN: (Goes over to garbage can and looks inside again. Walks away slowly, keeping garbage can in view)

MA: Don't tell me you have something else to do. Dishes come first!

YOUNG MAN: (Walks back to can, sticks head inside, moves back) Sounds like her. She must have followed me here. *(Turns in every direction looking for mother)* Ma, you here? Where are you? Stop fooling me.

MA: Marjorie will be home soon with the groceries, and the dishes still aren't done. I want you to do them before she gets home.

YOUNG MAN: (Goes back to can and kicks it hard) Tell Marjorie to go "f" herself. *(Walks away, then comes back. Puts can back in place)* I'm sorry. Ma, you hear me? I said, I'm sorry. *(Knocks on can as though it's a door)* Ma, you there?

MA: Of course I'm here. Where do you think I am, at home, waiting for you to do the dishes?

YOUNG MAN: (Desperate) I don't believe you. You're not here. I just left you at home screaming about how you had too much to do, how you couldn't stand to see me laying around listening to music when the house was such a mess. So I say a swear. And you yell, "Don't you talk to me like that, young man." And I say, "I didn't say it to *you.*" So I decide to go out, and you say, "Don't bother to come back until you're ready to do your share around here, without me asking."

MA: If your memory is so good how come you can't remember when you're supposed to do the dishes?

YOUNG MAN: If you weren't a queer, I wouldn't have any problems.

MA: I suppose you didn't do your homework yet, either?

YOUNG MAN: I'm going out.

MA: I want to know when you're coming home.

YOUNG MAN: Leave me alone. *(Kicks garbage can over)* Damn, I didn't mean it. I can't believe this. *(Gently puts can upright)* I don't know what I'm doing, acting like you're my mother. *(Mimes turning on radio. Popular song begins to play loudly. He moves around in a relaxed way in time to the music and also begins to groom his hair)*

MA: Turn down the music, I can't hear myself think.

YOUNG MAN: (Angrily turns off radio) Why can't you be like other mothers?

MA: Electricity costs money; don't leave your stereo on when you go out.

YOUNG MAN: *(Very upset)* What do you think it's like for me? I can't invite my friends over. What if they find out?

MA: If you cleaned up your room you could invite your friends over.

YOUNG MAN: Everyone knows, the landlord, the whole neighborhood. You two look like a couple of guys walking down the street. *(Lights dim. Young man exits)*

MA: *(Lighting change indicating evening. Yells to son offstage)* Please vacuum the living room; you dropped your Fritos all over it. *(Phone rings)* Hi Jan . . . Yeah, he's got a cold; went out without his jacket again . . . He just feels lonely; says he doesn't have any friends . . . I think Marjorie and I will stay home tonight, play a game with him or something.

YOUNG MAN: *(Lighting change indicating daytime. Enters slowly. Knocks gently on can)* Ma, you there? Ma. Some kids I know beat up this guy who hangs out on the streets, called him a fag, said he had AIDS. Ma, you hear me? *(Frustrated. Picks up garbage can and yells into it)* That's what's going to happen to me. They'll think I'm a queer 'cause you're a lezzie. *(Pause. Puts down can)* I should have stopped them, Ma. How can I stop them? I hate myself.

MA: You wanted to stop them, that's what matters. There was only one of you and a lot of them. Probably nothing you could do. Who I am, who you are, what others think; it's going to get easier as you get older, I promise.

YOUNG MAN: *(Pause. Takes deep breath. Begins again. Puts hands in pockets and looks down shyly)* Got almost all A's this quarter, Ma, and my English teacher really liked the sci-fi story I wrote.

MA: I'm really proud of you.

YOUNG MAN: I like this girl. But she's going out with a guy. He's older. She says she likes me better. Then this other girl who's been wanting me to ask her out—her friends told me—she asked me to go to the movies. I don't know what to do. *(Pause)*

Why can't I have a beer once in a while? Sometimes I'd just like to relax in front of the TV and drink a beer. My friend with the car, we don't drink or nothing, just ride around or go to the movies.

MA: I suppose we have to talk about safe sex and how to protect yourself. You can still get AIDS or get somebody pregnant.

YOUNG MAN: *(Embarrassed)* We had sex education in school.

MA: Just make sure you use condoms, latex ones. Oh, maybe not latex ones any more, some people are allergic. Never mind, I'll find out.

YOUNG MAN: *(Puts hands over ears and talks while mother talks about condoms)* You're just a garbage can. I'll pretend I didn't hear you. *(Crosses arms and whistles. Walks away slowly)* I don't talk to garbage cans. Jewish [change, if necessary, to indicate ethnic origin of the mother] ... mothers aren't supposed to be garbage cans. They're supposed to look pretty, cook nice meals, keep the house clean, iron clothes, sew on buttons. [Revise to reflect the normative constructs of motherhood for the particular ethnic group.]

MA: Thanks for doing all the laundry last night.

YOUNG MAN: *(Lifts lid off garbage can and fools around with it)* I needed to wash this shirt anyway.

MA: I thought you didn't talk to garbage cans.

YOUNG MAN: It's so much easier at my dad's house.

MA: That's not what you said the last time I talked to you after you and your father had another fight.

YOUNG MAN: Yeah. But he's getting *better*.

MA: What am *I*? Getting *worse*?

YOUNG MAN: Well, yeah. I used to think you were going to get back together with him, now I don't.

MA: Sounds like *you* are getting better.

YOUNG MAN: I'm going to join the army when I'm 18. I'll show you.

MA: Sometimes I wish you were a girl.

YOUNG MAN: Sometimes I wish you were a girl.

MA: Now we're even.

YOUNG MAN: You're hopeless.

MA: Never had more hope.

YOUNG MAN: You didn't used to get on my case about doing dishes and cleaning up my room and stuff, just since Marjorie moved in.

MA: I should have done it before.

YOUNG MAN: Well I liked it better the other way. *(Slams lid back on can)*

(Car horn sounds)

YOUNG MAN: Tell my dad I'll be right down, will you, Ma? He doesn't like it when I make him wait. *(Rushes around finishing getting dressed. Runs down stairs. Runs back. Car horn sounds again, more insistent)* Damn. *(Picks up garbage can and runs out of house)*

Questions for Classroom Discussion

The following questions should be helpful jumping-off places for classroom discussion. Students could spend some time writing in response to at least the first question and then have the opportunity to share their writing in small groups as well as in the large group. The other questions would also lend themselves to writing, but would also be very good discussion starters.

1. What did you think of the play and why?

2. What questions do you have about the play or the subject matter it touched upon?

3. What does the mother and son's relationship have in common with most other mothers and sons? What about mothers and daughters?

4. What seems unique about their relationship to lesbian- and gay-headed families?

5. What suggestions do you have for the mother and son to help them improve their relationship?

3

Multifaceted and Extended Dramas

These dramas have a variety of parts and can be extended over a longer period of time in order to delve more deeply into issues related to sexual orientation. Each drama explores a different aspect of lesbian and gay life. The first drama, *Sandy and Denny's Wedding*, views the institution of marriage and its effects on the individual lives of lesbians and gay people, their friends, and their family members. *Dealing with Heterosexism at Herbert Hoover High* revolves around a high school prom and explores the role of activist heterosexual allies in countering heterosexism. The third drama, *Homophobia and Racism at Pleasantville High*, examines homophobic and racial violence in a high school and how a community takes responsibility for reducing prejudice and creating a safer and more welcoming environment for everyone. It is a variation of the simple role-play outlined in Chapter 1.

This sequence of dramas corresponds to the process that many people follow in their transition from developing an awareness of lesbian, gay, bisexual, transsexual, transgender, and intersexual life to becoming change agents to help society embrace sexual and gender diversity.

The dramas also represent different degrees of complexity. Each can be done successfully over two or three sessions or days or shortened to one three-hour session. *Sandy and Denny's Wedding* is the only drama that has been developed for a three-day session. The complexity of the dramas, however, is not related to their lengths, but to the type of facilitation they require. The job of the facilitator is to guide participants through planned activities, giving them direct instructions when necessary, narrating a story, and enhancing the emotional and intellectual impact of the drama by stepping into role.

In this way, *Sandy and Denny's Wedding* is probably the most complex because it has the most complicated story line, demands both continuous narration of a story as well as facilitation in and out of role, and entails some complex role-playing on the part of the facilitator. It can be led by one facilitator but works best with two to three facilitators. The workshop's general purpose is to explore the wide range of views about lesbian and gay partnerships and marriage in both the straight and gay communities and to sensitize participants to the impact of homophobia and heterosexism on the lives of lesbian and gay couples. The three-day workshop is outlined in this section with suggestions for reducing it to a three-hour format.

The initial inspiration for this drama was a workshop I attended, led by British educational drama educator Gavin Bolton, in the summer of 1992 as part of New York University's Study Abroad Program in Educational Theater. Gavin was demonstrating one of his extended dramas based upon the Sleeping Beauty fairy tale. In his version of the story, Sleeping Beauty had just been born, and to escape a curse placed by a wicked fairy godmother on the child, the king and queen held a secret naming ceremony for her. The wicked fairy godmother found out about it anyhow, as wicked fairy godmothers are wont to do. When she entered (Gavin in role), I was standing on the outside edge of the group of invited guests. I will never forget my shock and embarrassment when that godmother tricked me into revealing the whereabouts of the innocent baby. As a result of this experience, I was better able to see life as full of surprises and reversals and drama as a vehicle for better understanding life's complexities. Homophobia, instead of the wicked fairy godmother, became the obstacle in my drama. It completely disrupts peoples' lives and cannot be ignored.

The second drama can be easily facilitated by one person in role throughout. The drama was inspired by a novel by Aaron Fricke, *Reflections of a Rock Lobster* (1981), about a young man coming out in high school and taking his boyfriend to the prom. But it goes beyond this story line to explore the importance of individual activism in lessening heterosexism and homophobia in schools. The drama also explores the work of gay/straight alliances in schools, the role of heterosexual allies, and symbols of queer culture that are not readily understood by people outside the culture.

In the third drama the facilitator(s) is also in role but sometimes acts simply as a narrator guiding participants through each stage of the drama. The roles the facilitator plays in this drama are fictional composite characters that represent three different groups of people who are deeply affected by homophobia: sexual minority students, LGBT teachers, and parents. The roles and the parts the participants play are derived from an article from the *New York Times* by Evelyn Nieves (1999) about a violent attack on a gay student in a high school thirty miles north of San Francisco. The drama, like the article, makes connections between racism and homophobia and stresses the need for schools to address all incidents of bias and to work to reduce all forms of prejudice in the communities they serve.

All the dramas can be conducted successfully with fifteen to forty participants and are designed to help participants examine their own biases, feel the effects of prejudice against sexual minorities, and explore ways to reduce homophobia in society. Some of the work in these drama activities is closely guided within the framework of a story, and some of it is self-directed by the participants. What ultimately happens in the story as it unfolds is determined, in large part, by the participants.

The description of each workshop in this chapter begins with a summary of the story to familiarize teachers with the events of the drama in the order in which they unfold. The story is then elaborated upon, section by section, to help teachers facilitate these dramas easily in their own classrooms. Samples of facilitated dialogue are included to give teachers more of a flavor of what it is possible to do within the parameters of facilitator-in-role. These dialogue samples are only intended as examples of what may be possible. Following each section are content and drama goals to coincide with each part of the drama. Occasionally, references are also included to help teachers increase their own content knowledge about a particular area, or to suggest ways of drawing upon a wider knowledge base in the drama itself through the use of artifacts.

Sandy and Denny's Wedding

Suggested Readings

Lambda Legal Defense and Education Fund, Marriage Project, www.lambdalegal.org

Gay and Lesbian Alliance Against Defamation—GLAADLines, www.glaad.org

Same-Sex Marriage: Pro and Con—A Reader, by Andrew Sullivan

Sappho Goes to Law School, by Ruthann Robson

Local newspaper articles

Materials

Envelope with invitation

Art materials to create wedding gift

Role cards

Kazoos and other celebratory noisemakers, confetti, etc.

Lyrics of "The Anniversary Song," by Al Jolson and Saul Chaplin (see appendix pp. 115–16)

Summary

Participants examine the complexities of same-sex marriage from various view-points, as LGBT people who have decided to marry and as their friends and family members, both supportive and hostile.

One Saturday morning you wake up and go to the mailbox to see if anything interesting has arrived for you. A small square card in an envelope looks intriguing. You open it and read it aloud. It is an invitation to Sandy Minsky and Denny Booth's wedding and you have been asked to RSVP. The invitation is somewhat puzzling, so you decide to phone a close friend or relative to talk over your feelings.

You and most of the others who received an invitation decide to attend. The couple has asked that everyone bring a wedding gift that symbolizes the couple's relationship to each other and your hopes for their future.

One person who was invited to the wedding, however, decides not to go. While everyone is making the gifts, Aunt Lena or Uncle Larry arrives. S/he accuses the wedding guests who are just finishing their gifts of being hypocrites and liars, and just as bad as the couple who s/he feels are making a mockery of the sacred institution of marriage by marrying someone of the same sex. Aunt Lena/Uncle Larry leaves and some of the guests decide to revise their gifts to the couple, based upon the angry relative's response.

At the couple's request, the wedding guests, who represent close relatives, distant relatives, coworkers or fellow students, and close friends, create the wedding ceremony. During the ceremony, each group, beginning with close family members and ending with close friends, ritually present their gifts, explaining the symbolic meaning of each gift they have created.

All the guests are socializing and enjoying themselves at the reception when Aunt Lena/Uncle Larry arrives. S/he brings a special gift for the couple. It is a bitter song s/he has written especially for the occasion. After the song, s/he departs abruptly. Feeling strongly about what has just happened, the guests create a landscape of Aunt Lena/Uncle Larry's life, trying to understand what has influenced her/him.

It is now ten years later and life has not been a bed of roses for Sandy and Denny. As a matter of fact, they have decided to split up. Their friends and family try to figure out why this has happened.

And, as can be expected, Aunt Lena/Uncle Larry arrives to say, "I told you so. If everyone had just listened to me, there would not be so much heartache now." This is the last straw for the people who have followed Sandy and Denny's relationship closely and who wanted the best for them. They confront Aunt Lena/Uncle Larry on her/his homophobia for the first time.

First Day

Introduction

The facilitator introduces the topic of lesbian and gay marriage by asking participants who have some knowledge about the struggle of lesbian and gay people to gain marriage rights to share what they know. However, the facilitator needs to let participants know that through the drama workshop they will be exploring this topic in a different way than some of them have done before, this time as people who have something at stake. After the workshop the facilitator and participants will share specific information about the present status of lesbian and gay marriage and domestic partnership struggles in the United States and in other parts of the world. (The appendix contains material from Lambda Legal Defense and Education Fund's Marriage Project. The website is updated continuously.)

Providing the participants with a general introduction to working through drama (see the introductory chapter for suggestions) is also important, including some reasons that the workshop examines this issue through drama. Other reasons will become apparent to participants during the course of the workshop. To prepare people for the drama, it is important let participants know, that they will be expected to step into a variety of roles, with assistance, and to interact with others in role. Participants should also have a chance to ask questions about the process or to share experiences, good or bad, they might have had with drama. This often helps others clarify and articulate what their own apprehensions might be.

Objectives

To introduce the content area, facilitators will find it useful to become familiar with different arguments put forth in gay and straight communities in support of and against lesbian and gay marriages. This issue, like the issue of gays in the military, has become a battleground that is constantly in flux between advocates for lesbian and gay civil rights and right-wing forces, led by the religious right, who continue to claim that homosexuality is a sin and/or that gay people have a sickness that can be cured. Educators wishing to work with the issue of gay marriage need to keep up-to-date on the latest developments.

The Lambda Legal Defense and Education Fund's Marriage Project and Gay and Lesbian Alliance Against Defamation's GLAADLines, both of which can be accessed through the World Wide Web, contain up-to-date and background articles that will give facilitators and students an abundance of information about the status of the struggle of sexual minorities for the right to marry. *Same-Sex Marriage: Pro and Con—A Reader* (Sullivan 1997) offers a history of the debate about lesbian and gay marriage and the central arguments pro and con from both a straight and gay perspective.

Asking people to speak about their fears in relation to drama helps others clarify and articulate what their own apprehensions might be. Better to get them on the table than to have people sit and worry and resist participation.

The Invitation

The narrator begins to tell a story, setting the scene by describing the weather, the time of day, and what the participants have been doing, and then directs them to go to the mailbox to see if the mail they had been expecting has arrived. The mail they had been expecting is not there, but something unexpected is. It is a small square envelope.

The facilitator gives each participant an envelope and asks everyone to read aloud the enclosed invitation. It reads: "You are invited to Sandy Minsky and Denny Booth's wedding. It will be held at the Overlook Pavilion at Buena Vista Park, Sunday, June 3, at noon. RSVP."

Objectives

The first activity is designed to bring the participants into the drama immediately through a hazily defined role as someone who receives an invitation to a wedding. This initial role-play, or icebreaker, helps prepare the participants for the next phases of the drama, in which they will be asked to evolve into more fleshed-out characters with stronger points of view.

The invitation is an artifact that concretely dramatizes the story and helps create belief in the fiction being developed. Reading the invitation out loud is ritualistic and brings everyone into the moment through a shared experience. It also introduces the theme of marriage and gives legitimacy to the wedding couple's relationship.

Note that the people getting married have generic names and cannot be identified as either female or male. Because gender is not indicated on the invitation, and the first names can indicate either female or male gender, some participants will assume this is an invitation to a hetero-sexual couple's wedding, some will assume that two men are getting married, and some that the wedding is for two women.

The Phone Call

The narrator then tells the participants to make a phone call to a close friend or relative to talk about the invitation.

The facilitator asks participants to form pairs with someone nearby and decide who will call and who will respond. The respondent must go along with the conversation the caller begins. The facilitator also can assign roles of caller and respondent to the pairs.

Objectives

The first interactions in role are often the hardest. Working in pairs to discuss their feelings about Sandy and Denny's wedding is another ice-breaking activity that helps the participants gain some comfort with the issues. Using exploratory talk to share their ideas with someone else helps prepare participants for going further into the drama in the larger group.

Participants begin to define their roles during the phone call and practice important intrapersonal and interpersonal skills. The person in the pair who initiates the conversation imagines and initiates a particular narrative. The responder joins someone else's creative narrative and becomes a partner in that fiction.

Create Wedding Gifts

Continuing the story, the narrator tells the participants that they have all decided to go to the wedding, no matter what they are feeling about it, and that this is the first time they have ever been invited to a lesbian or gay wedding. The narrator explains they will be giving the couple a symbolic wedding gift representing the couple's relationship and their hopes for the couple's future.

The facilitator now asks the pairs to join with one or two other pairs, depending upon the size of the group. In all, the participants should be divided into four groups. Each group is instructed to first decide the gender/sex of the couple. (There are no right or wrong answers. It is just important to make sure that the group has either reached a consensus on this question or that everyone is at least willing to go along with a particular decision.)

The facilitator then asks each group to create a representation of their symbolic wedding gift, first by having a go-around within the group to make a list of everyone's ideas for the gift, and then democratically selecting the idea that works best for everyone. Every member of the group contributes to the gift. It can resemble an everyday object but must primarily be a symbolic representation of their feelings about the couple and their wishes for their future. The gift must have some type of concrete representation and can take the form of a mural or sculpture or other object. Participants use markers, paper, string, tape, glue, scissors, and other art materials to create their gifts.

Objectives

Those who assumed the couple is heterosexual will now have a chance to revise their idea.

Some participants may feel inadequate or competitive when asked to create the gift. It is useful to remind people that they don't need to be artists to do this activity. Whatever people create is symbolic and represents whatever they tell us it means.

This activity is designed to bring the participants into the story tangibly, giving them all something concrete to make and ownership of what they have created.

The creation of the initial gift is a cooperative learning activity in which people begin to form trusting working relationships with one another, a key to the success of the workshop. The guidelines include the following: everyone must participate, everyone must listen to each group member, the group must incorporate everyone's ideas, everyone must take turns, and the group must make decisions that everyone can live with.

In this stage of the drama, participants begin to explore their own and each other's ideas about marriage in general, its positive and negative aspects, and how the institution of marriage specifically relates to gay couples, or how gay couples relate to it. Throughout the workshop, participants are given more and more opportunity to speak about things that many of them have never spoken about before. This lack of vocabulary and/or voice tends to be a strong barrier in doing effective antihomophobia education. A key to doing this work effectively is to give participants opportunities to interact with the new material they are learning, or the new feelings that are being evoked throughout the workshop, as well as many opportunities to give voice to their concerns.

Aunt Lena/Uncle Larry Enters

Once the participants seem close to completing their gifts, the narrator gets everyone's attention and announces that one person who was invited decided not to go to the wedding.

A facilitator in role as Aunt Lena/Uncle Larry enters. (The facilitator should be comfortable in his or her role. Some may find it easier to maintain their gender identity, while others may see this role as an opportunity to cross gender lines.) S/he goes up to the different groups as they work, questioning them about the gifts they are creating.

After seeing what people are doing, s/he addresses the participants as a group, accusing them of hypocrisy and lying. S/he claims that the participants indicated on the phone with her/him that they were very unhappy with the marriage and did not feel it was moral. She accuses them all of being just as immoral as the couple. Aunt Lena/Uncle Larry exits as s/he murmurs something about making a mockery of the institution of marriage.

Objectives

Aunt Lena/Uncle Larry's entrance gives the participants an opportunity to discuss with an audience outside their group what they have created and why.

There are many things that Aunt Lena/Uncle Larry can say here, depending on the experience of the participants of the group. S/he could talk in the voice of a very religious person, but not from the viewpoint of a particular religious denomination. It is important to play this role respectfully and not to target a particular religion. S/he may play the role from the point of view of someone who has a conservative secular background. S/he may be conservative politically. S/he may have had a traumatic experience that has shaped her/his worldview. A combination of several of these elements may determine what s/he says and does. At no time should Aunt Lena/Uncle Larry be portrayed stereotypically. S/he represents a real voice in society. S/he is someone bound by tradition and afraid of change, who may not realize how much hurt s/he is causing or how s/he has incorporated into her/himself the hatred in the society around her/him. S/he does not necessarily have to be someone who can change.

The basic purpose of the character of Aunt Lena/Uncle Larry is to introduce conflict into the drama and the issue of homophobia and heterosexism from outside the group. Introducing it from outside the group makes it safer for those who are influenced by similar prejudices within the group and those who have been hurt by similar prejudices in others. Introducing this character helps participants to continue to work despite their own discomfort and without putting them on the spot. Gavin Bolton says that the dramatic purpose of introducing a conflict such as this is to "skew" the drama (1992a), showing that even a happy occasion like a wedding isn't always bright and rosy. Skewing also enriches the experience of the participants, making it more realistic and giving them more of an opportunity to use their imaginations. But its greatest benefit in a workshop such as this is to help the participants reach a deeper level of experience and meaning.

Discussion

After Aunt Lena/Uncle Larry's emotional outburst, the facilitator asks people to finish up their gifts and then to move into a circle to talk about what happened from the point of view of their characters. Some questions the facilitator might ask to get the discussion going: What gender did your group assign to Sandy and Denny and why? How did you feel about what Aunt Lena/Uncle Larry said? What other feelings came up for you that you would like to talk about?

Objectives

Participants are asked to step out of role for this discussion to reflect on the roles they have played in the drama so far. This is the first time the participants will have the opportunity to discuss Aunt Lena/Uncle Larry's prejudices, to talk about how it felt to be confronted by those feelings, and to look at similar feelings they might have or might have experienced. For some participants, this may be the first chance they have to discuss what a lesbian or gay relationship is and what it might be like for lesbians and gay men to deal with a prejudiced relative or prejudice in other parts of their lives.

Revise Gifts

After the discussion, the facilitator asks participants to return to their groups and asks each group to choose one role card. The role cards identify particular people in the couple's life whom each group will represent—close family, distant family, friends or colleagues from work or school, and close friends. The facilitator asks people, for the first time, to think about who they specifically are within that group, to discuss their characters with the others in their group, and to try to achieve as much diversity in terms of point of view and background within the groups as possible.

Once the group members are clear about who they are and who they represent in the couple's lives, the facilitator asks them to go back to the gift they created and revise it, if necessary, depending upon the new roles they are playing and how they feel after reflecting on Aunt Lena/Uncle Larry's intervention. Are they still satisfied with the gift, or do they want to make changes? The facilitator reminds the groups to pay attention to one another and listen carefully to what other people are saying, but also to try to be clear about their own thoughts and feelings and try to figure out how to make a decision that best reflects everyone's interests.

Objectives

Stepping into concrete roles at this point in the drama asks people to rethink and perhaps revise their first ideas. Working through a more concrete character gives participants more of a chance to voice doubts about the rights or desirability of lesbian and gay people getting married, from their own perspectives or those of other people in society.

From a drama perspective, stepping into these roles gives the participants more of a context from which to respond with their whole beings to events in the story as they unfold.

Plan Ceremony

The facilitator then explains how the participants will create the ceremony. Each group first chooses two people from their group to represent the couple. The group that is close family will create the beginning portion, distant family the next, friends from work the next, and close friends will create the last part. Each group is to include the presentation of the gift as part of a ritual, making sure that the couple understands all of its symbolic meaning. The ritual should combine a variety of forms, such as movement, dance, music, and poetry.

Conduct Ceremony

When the groups have completed their plans, the narrator announces that the ceremony is about to begin. Everyone throws confetti and plays kazoos or other musical instruments in celebration. The facilitator asks each group to introduce themselves and to make sure that the other wedding guests, who may be asked to involve themselves in another group's ritual, understand what they are supposed to do. The groups facilitate the entire ceremony themselves.

Objectives

The wedding ceremony gives the participants a chance to attain a deep level of feeling. It also gives them the chance to experience the social and personal significance of lesbian and gay marriage, whether forbidden or sanctioned, and what it can be like for lesbian and gay people to create their own rituals and ceremonies. (Some churches and synagogues now perform standard ceremonies for lesbian and gay couples or ceremonies that have been adapted for same-sex couples.) In the process participants will be thinking about how these ceremonies might compare to traditional wedding ceremonies and the type of ceremony they might choose if they were lesbian or gay people getting married.

Reflection

Participants write about the feelings and thoughts they had during the unfolding of the drama. What stood out for them? What was comfortable and uncomfortable? What might they do differently? How did they feel during the planning and performance of the ceremony? What did it mean to them? They then share at least portions of what they wrote with the whole group.

Objectives

It is important to leave plenty of time for writing and discussion. This can be the richest part of the workshop; it is where synthesis happens. The drama itself can be viewed as merely the spark that ignites learning. Asking participants to write about their thoughts and feelings gives them time to recall different thoughts and feelings they have had so far and helps prepare each participant to contribute something to the discussion. It is important for the reflection time to be long enough to accommodate everyone, giving each person a chance to share a thought or feeling, and giving everyone who needs to a chance to debrief or work through a difficult or intense moment that occurred for him during the drama.

Second Day

The Wedding Reception

The narrator now situates the guests at the wedding reception. Guests introduce themselves to people they don't know, perhaps asking questions about

group members' participation in the ceremony, learning more about each other, about the couple, socializing. The couple thank the guests for their gifts and ask questions, if necessary, to further clarify the gifts' symbolic meanings.

Objectives
This is a time for participants to resituate themselves in the drama, learn more about how others have constructed the wedding couple, and understand the meaning people gave to different aspects of the ceremony.

Aunt Lena/Uncle Larry Enters

After the guests have a chance to socialize, the narrator announces that a guest has arrived who originally was not going to come. Aunt Lena/Uncle Larry enters and says s/he has changed her/his mind about attending the reception and announces s/he has brought a wedding gift for the couple. It is a special song s/he has written.

Objectives
Skewing the drama again, when everyone is congratulating everyone else and feeling relatively good about her role and the marriage ceremony, brings the participants back to the tenacity and pervasiveness of homophobia, how deep-rooted it is, and how we need to address it continuously.

Write Wedding Songs

The facilitator asks the participants to return to their groups, step out of the roles they were in previously, and step into role as Aunt Lena/Uncle Larry. The facilitator gives each group the music to "The Anniversary Song" with room to write alternative words. People who are familiar with it sing the original version. Every group is asked to rewrite two lines of the song in role as Aunt Lena/Uncle Larry. While everyone is writing, Aunt Lena/Uncle Larry walks around, making sure that her/his feelings are being represented as accurately as possible in the lyrics.

Sing Wedding Songs

The narrator asks for the presentation of the song and Aunt Lena/Uncle Larry sings along with each group. At the end of the singing, Aunt Lena/Uncle Larry makes a brief statement about how at last her/his sentiments are being heard and then quickly exits.

Objectives

The objective of this exercise is to involve the participants more thoroughly in the dramatic conflict. After expressing mostly positive feelings during the ceremony, the participants now experience contrasting feelings—Aunt Lena/Uncle Larry's anger and pain. They are compelled to express the hatred, anger, and fear Aunt Lena/Uncle Larry feels, perhaps giving voice to some of their own fears and prejudices or those they have experienced or noticed in others. But, because they are in role as Aunt Lena/Uncle Larry, they may feel safer expressing negative feelings. It is very important in prejudice reduction work to give participants an opportunity to look inside themselves and bring to light feelings and ideas they may have that may even be unconscious. Stepping into role as a homophobic character also helps the participants empathize and learn more about the psychology of a person who fears or hates lesbian and gay people. In this way, they may develop empathy for the homophobic person, just as they are developing empathy for the lesbian or gay people. Such empathy can make it easier for people to communicate more effectively with people whose views are so negative and different from their own.

Create and Share Landscapes

The facilitator asks people to step out of role for this activity and to work alone. Each person is asked to create an imaginary landscape of Aunt Lena/Uncle Larry's life, using whatever objects are in the room or in their pockets or bags. They choose one of the objects to represent Aunt Lena/Uncle Larry and have her/him move through the landscape they have created as s/he has moved through her/his life. They are asked to write about the landscapes, share them in small groups, and ask one another questions about the process each person went through to create his landscape.

Objectives

This activity is designed to give Aunt Lena/Uncle Larry's fear and prejudice a context and make the character more three-dimensional.

Here the participants have a chance to reflect on the intense experiences they have just had and distance themselves a little from the uncomfortable role they just played as Aunt Lena/Uncle Larry. The overall objective here is to get the participants to think about the possible causes of Lena/Larry's attitudes and the roots of individual prejudice. They will need to get inside the character of the homophobe in order to eventually be successful in standing up to her/him. The violent reactions of homophobic people in families and in the general society to sexual minorities, and the pervasive media coverage they get, often make them seem ubiquitous and impossible to counteract. This activity begins the process of making homophobia more real. It increases the potential for eliminating it through intensive prejudice reduction work, lessening its effects by increasing one's distance from it, or keeping it under control through community education and law enforcement.

Reflection

Participants write and reflect on the second day's workshop. Prompts posed by the facilitator might include the following: Compare how you felt on each day and what you thought about. Think about what it was like to step into role as Aunt Lena/Uncle Larry and then to create the landscapes. What questions arose during the second day of the workshop?

Objectives

Asking participants to reflect on the second day's activities and compare them to the first day helps people look at more dimensions of homophobia, what causes it, and how it hurts so many people. It also gives participants a chance to ask questions or work through feelings generated by the second day of the workshop in which they stepped into homophobic roles themselves and developed some degree of empathy for someone with homophobic beliefs. Stepping into the shoes of someone whom we do not respect or whose values we abhor can be very difficult emotionally, but in a supportive environment this work can be enlightening and useful, particularly for someone who wants to make a difference in reducing prejudice.

Third Day

The Breakup

The third day begins with the narrator setting the scene: It's ten years later. Life has been hard for Sandy and Denny. In fact, they have decided to split up.

The facilitator asks people to divide up into different groups of anywhere from four to eight members, to create images of the couple using only their bodies. Each group is asked to be responsible for creating two images or tableaux. The guidelines are similar to those of the last group—everyone in the group becomes part of the tableaux and everyone's ideas are taken into consideration, even if they cannot all be adopted. At least two people in each tableau play the couple. One image should represent a personal reason that led to the couple's breakup; the other should represent how society may have made it difficult for the couple to remain together. Participants may use some words along with these images—two sentences at most.

Objectives

The purpose of this turn in the plot, like introducing Aunt Lena/ Uncle Larry, is to give the participants another unanticipated obstacle and draw them further into the tension of the story. The breakup is also designed to show that lesbian and gay couples, like heterosexual couples, may or may not stay together forever. In this portion of the workshop, the issues of monogamy and non-monogamy may be introduced or reintroduced, along with other sexuality and relationship issues that are concerns both in the gay community and in the society at large.

This is an opportunity for the participants to play the roles of the lesbian or gay couple and to try to see their daily lives from a queer perspective. It is designed to show that lesbian and gay people have some of the same problems and issues as everyone else as well as some different issues, and, in addition, they have to contend with widespread homophobia in society.

Asking participants to change groups gives them opportunities for working with others in the workshop, increasing their exposure to different perspectives and giving them opportunities to practice the cooperative group skills they have been developing throughout the workshop.

Present Tableaux

After each group presents its tableaux, the narrator asks Sandy and Denny to explain the reasons for their breakup to the others. The narrator encourages their friends and family members to ask questions to make sure they fully understand what happened.

To develop the story through an aesthetic lens, the facilitator also asks the groups and other participants for ideas for making the tableaux stronger or

clearer. The groups can then revise the tableaux based upon the feedback they received. Participants can suggest that individuals make larger gestures, add more sound or words, use more space, add or change movements, and so on.

Objectives

Presenting, discussing, and analyzing the images they have created in the tableaux helps everyone better understand the pressures on the sexual minority couple. This is also an opportunity to increase the dramatic tension through theater techniques. In this process, participants begin to better understand the relationship between theater and life and how theater can highlight different aspects of life by intensifying particular events and bringing them under greater scrutiny.

Confront Homophobia

Once the groups have presented their enhanced images, Aunt Lena/Uncle Larry reenters. S/he tells the group that this is just what s/he predicted and that if people had listened to her/him, this terrible thing would not have happened. The drama is now placed into the hands of the participants, who respond to Aunt Lena/Uncle Larry. If nothing happens immediately, the narrator can coax them a bit with questions or comments, such as "Are you just going to let her/him get away with this?" or "Isn't it time that someone stand up to this person?"

Objectives

This is the moment that Gavin Bolton calls "pushing the button" (1992a), the place where the participants are provoked to determine what happens next. In this section the participants finally have the chance to confront Aunt Lena/Uncle Larry, her/his bigotry, her/his pain, and the pain s/he is causing others. They may tackle whom s/he represents societally, they may decide to expel her/him. It is really up to them. At first everyone will just be given a chance to respond to her/him, perhaps confronting homophobia directly for the first time—a moment many people greatly fear.

If their confrontation of Aunt Lena/Uncle Larry does not go far enough, or not enough people participate, the workshop leaders can suggest that participants choose a dramatic activity that will bring them one step further. At this point, the workshop leader is mainly a resource for dramatic strategies to help the participants reach goals they have defined for themselves.

Hot Seat Lena/Larry (optional)

Depending upon time available and if the confrontation of Aunt Lena/Uncle Larry does not go very far, the workshop facilitator(s) can take the drama one step further. It is important, however, to keep what happens next in the hands of the participants.

If they decide to continue, the narrator lets the workshop participants know that they are not yet done with their work in confronting homophobia. It is important that they get underneath the confrontation and become more effective at neutralizing homophobic forces. To do this they will use a drama strategy called "Hot Seating" (Neelands 1990, 28). One person from each group will volunteer to be Aunt Lena/Uncle Larry and will sit in a row facing the rest of the group. The others, back in the roles of their original groups, will question Aunt Lena/Uncle Larry about her/his prejudiced attitudes and behaviors. In response, Aunt Lena/Uncle Larry will draw upon the landscapes s/he created. In questioning Aunt Lena/Uncle Larry, the participants as the couple and the couple's friends and family members will both uncover the causes of homophobia as well as challenge the perpetrator's bigoted attitudes and behaviors.

See Jonothan Neelands' *Structuring Drama Work* (1990) for further ideas and drama strategies that might be useful in this portion of the drama.

Closure

Participants are asked to spend some time writing about whatever questions remain for them or what stood out for them in the workshop. Other prompts for writing and discussion might be about changes in their thoughts and feelings about lesbian and gay marriage and relationships as a result of the workshop, or about their feelings about standing up to homophobia in relatives and in social institutions. A significant amount of time should be spent sharing their writing and thoughts in the large group.

Objectives

The purpose of this final reflective writing and discussion is to give participants a chance to express their personal responses to the workshop. It is an opportunity to see what participants accomplished and what issues they avoided or missed. The writing and discussion also empowers participants to think about ways they might revise such a workshop to better suit their own needs.

Often the discussion after an intensive workshop like this is highly charged, and it is a good idea to have participants first explore their experiences and reactions by writing about them, which helps to warm up people for discussion. Then they can more easily air their thoughts, fears, and ideas and demonstrate the comfort they have gained about working with complex aspects of gay and lesbian relationships and society's resistance to validating these relationships.

Three-Day Workshop Outline

I. First Day
   A. Introduction
   B. The Invitation
   C. The Phone Call
   D. Create Wedding Gifts
   E. Aunt Lena/Uncle Larry Enters
   F. Discussion
   G. Revise Gifts
   H. Plan Ceremoney
   I. Conduct Ceremony
   J. Reflection

II. Second Day
   A. The Wedding Reception
   B. Aunt Lena/Uncle Larry Enters
   C. Write Wedding Songs
   D. Sing Wedding Songs
   E. Create and Share Landscapes
   F. Reflection

III. Third Day
   A. The Breakup
   B. Present Tableaux
   C. Confront Homophobia
   D. Hot Seat Lena/Larry
   E. Closure

Three-Hour Workshop Outline

The three-hour workshop consolidates many features of the three-day workshop. Because a great deal of time is needed for drawing in a workshop such as this, the wedding gift is transformed into a symbolic movement piece choreographed by each group and composed of a movement contribution from each group member.

Less time is also spent warming up participants, getting beneath Aunt Lena/Uncle Larry's homophobia, and exploring personal and social dimensions of the effects of homophobia. There will also be less time to give participants experience with confronting homophobia, and writing and reflection time will be limited to the end of the entire drama experience.

A. Introduction

B. The Invitation

C. Create Wedding Gifts

D. Aunt Lena/Uncle Larry Enters

E. Plan and Perform Ceremony

F. The Wedding Reception

G. Aunt Lena/Uncle Larry Enters

H. Write and Sing Wedding Songs

I. The Breakup

J. Confront Homophobia

K. Closure

Dealing with Heterosexism at Herbert Hoover High

Suggested Readings

Confessions of a Rock Lobster, by Aaron Fricke

Gay Straight Alliances: A Student Guide, Massachusetts Department of Education

School's Out: The Impact of Gay and Lesbian Issues on America's Schools, by Dan Woog

Supporting Youth: Their Education and Survival, video produced by In the Life

Materials

Poster board and markers

Lyrics and music to song, "We Kiss in a Shadow" (see appendix)

Summary

This drama explores the heterosexist underpinnings of the high school prom. It takes place in an organizational setting and demonstrates how activists, in this case a heterosexual ally of a queer student, can be an agent for social change.

The Gay/Straight Alliance (GSA) at Herbert Hoover High School has been boycotting the school prom for the past three years, since a lesbian couple was physically attacked and thrown out of the prom party for dancing together. The alliance declared the official school prom a heterosexist nightmare and began holding its own graduation parties at a protected location.

This year, a heterosexual student on the prom committee whose lesbian friends refused to attend the official prom is determined to make the prom celebration more welcoming and safe for LGBT students. She brings the committee's draft prom fliers to the Gay/Straight Alliance for approval.

The alliance makes suggestions, which the committee incorporates into the fliers. Copies are posted all over the school. In response, the PTA meets to raise concerns about the fliers. Students from the GSA and the prom committee attend the PTA meeting to answer those concerns.

Encouraged by the organizing, members of the Gay/Straight Alliance decide to attend the prom. Everyone sings and dances to the last song of the evening, one requested by the alliance, "We Kiss in the Shadow," from the Rogers and Hammerstein musical *South Pacific*.

Introduction

The facilitator prepares the participants for their work through drama by talking with them about drama, the difference between drama and theater, and what will be expected of them (see introduction to previous drama). The facilitator explains that in this drama she will guide the participants directly and also in role.

The facilitator also introduces the content of the workshop. Ideally, participants will have read the article about gay/straight alliances (GSAs) in *School's Out* by Dan Woog (1995, 268–79), as well as a book like Aaron Fricke's *Confessions of a Rock Lobster* (1981), or a story or essay from one of a number of anthologies that discuss the effects of heterosexist institutions and cultural events on the lives of queer youth, and/or seen a relevant video such as *Supporting Youth: Their Education and Survival* (2000). The facilitator should be up-to-date about gay/straight alliances and what they do locally and in other parts of the country. The website of the Gay, Lesbian, Straight Education Network (GLSEN) contains a great deal of local and national information about GSAs (www.glsen.org). Participants in the workshop may also have personal experiences with these groups that they may want to share.

Student Council Creates Prom Flier

The facilitator, in role as the prom committee ally, welcomes everyone to the work session to get the prom fliers ready. She brings out markers and paper and everyone gets to work. Students break down into groups of four to brainstorm and create the fliers.

After the groups complete the fliers, she raises concerns that they may not be welcoming enough to convince LGBT students to attend. This gives prom committee members the opportunity to express their points of view about the GSA. In response, the ally talks about the history of the prom and how it has excluded LGBT students and made it necessary for them to hold their own celebration. She points out that the LGBT prom does not even receive funding from the school because it is not an official school activity.

Objectives

This exercise establishes the setting and the point of view of a particular group of high school students. The purpose of the flier is to give the drama concreteness and help participants feel ownership of something they have created. Working in groups helps the participants build community and group belief. In role as someone else, participants have opportunities to voice antigay feelings, either their own or what they have heard from others. Bringing such feelings and thoughts to the surface is a necessary step in the process of reexamining and reducing prejudice.

Meeting of Gay/Straight Alliance

The facilitator, continuing in role, now comes before the Gay/Straight Alliance and thanks them for meeting with her. The alliance members discuss their experience with heterosexism and homophobia in the school. She then presents the fliers the committee has created and asks the alliance if they feel the fliers would help LGBT students feel more welcome at the prom this year.

Objectives

The major conflict as well as the theme of the drama are introduced. Stepping into the shoes of les/bi/gay/trans students, participants use their imaginations to draw upon what they already know about discrimination against sexual minorities in high schools, which helps participants develop empathy and prepare themselves to learn more. This step also enhances the narrative with experiences from the point of view of sexual minority students.

Revision of Flier

The facilitator then asks members of the alliance to revise the original fliers to make them more LGBT–friendly. After the participants revise the fliers, the facilitator asks the group to take up the question of whether or not to continue having a separate prom.

Objectives
Participants have the opportunity to use their imaginations to problem solve about an issue with which most of them have had little experience. They must step into the shoes of LGBT students in order to imagine ways in which school activities can recognize and welcome the participation of those who have previously felt excluded.

Post Fliers

The facilitator as narrator explains that in two days the revised flier was posted all over school. Participants post new fliers around the room. The facilitator announces that the fliers' posting has prompted an emergency meeting of the PTA.

Objectives
Posting the fliers gives participants a sense of completion as well as an opportunity to move around, have gay-positive materials on the walls, and experience a bit of what it might be like to make the physical environment of a school reflect all its students.

PTA Meeting

The narrator welcomes parents and teachers to the PTA meeting, summarizing why the meeting was called, saying that people were concerned about the new prom fliers all over the building and some new curriculum initiatives at the school that address issues of sexual orientation. The facilitator then asks everyone to form groups in which participants can raise their concerns. The groups write their concerns on newsprint sheets and post them. The facilitator encourages the groups to raise all points of view on their sheets, not just the ones that are most commonly heard.

When they are through, the facilitator divides the group in half. One half becomes students. The facilitator welcomes the students to the meeting and has them read the sheets that are posted and address the concerns raised by the parents and teachers, this time from the students' perspectives.

Objectives

At the meeting the participants have the opportunity to listen to different opinions and articulate what they imagine are the viewpoints of parents and teachers in the community about lesbian and gay issues in the high school. Breaking parents and teachers into small groups gives everyone a chance to be heard, and participants gain exposure to a wide range of opinions in the community without focusing only on negative reactions. Participants in roles as students then have a chance to respond to both negative and positive feelings about the changes in the school.

The Prom

The facilitator announces that the awaited night is finally here and participants, in pairs as lesbian, gay, bisexual, and transgendered students, are on their way to the prom. The facilitator has each participant turn to the person nearest him, who will be his partner, and asks the pairs to close their eyes and imagine how they look, what they are wearing, their hairstyles, their demeanors, how their lovers look. The facilitator also asks them to think about how they are feeling and what is on their minds and then to share their feelings and thoughts with each other.

Objectives

Stepping into the shoes of lesbian and gay students, participants are better able to understand their feelings, joys, and insecurities. Even experiencing the discomfort of stepping across gender boundaries, as some students will do in becoming members of same-sex couples, will help participants understand more of the complexities of LGBT issues. (This is another situation where nervous laughter and acting out could make it difficult for the students to stay in role. The facilitator can assist by reminding students to focus on their new roles and the importance of stepping into someone else's shoes.)

The Last Dance

The narrator announces the last dance of the night. It is the 1949 song titled "We Kiss in a Shadow," from the Rogers and Hammerstein musical *South Pacific*. It is a song about how two people feel who are involved in an interracial relationship in a time period when this is not acceptable. The facilitator gives out the words to the song and everyone is invited to sing and dance to it.

Objectives

Although this song is decades old, it still captures the cultural phenomenon of the closet as well as the liberation LGBT people feel when they begin to open the closet door. Like all Broadway musicals, this show catered to two different audiences, one ostensibly heterosexual, and one for those "in the life," that is, homosexual (Miller 1998). Many of Broadway's scriptwriters, songwriters, and actors were and are members of sexual minorities (Douglas 1999; Holden 1999). This particular song, through its text and subtext, also links homophobia to racism, an important issue to discuss in the reflection period following the drama.

Reflection

Participants will spend a few minutes writing down the thoughts and feelings they had at each point in the drama—what they enjoyed, what made them uncomfortable, what they learned. After writing, participants share the major points that stood out for them with the whole group.

Objectives

Thinking about the feelings and thoughts they experienced throughout the course of the drama can help participants identify areas of discomfort that they still need to work on and areas in which they feel confident taking more of a stand against homophobia.

It Can Happen Here: Homophobia and Racism at Pleasantville High

Suggested Readings

"Attacks on a Gay Teen-Ager Prompt Outrage and Soul-Searching," by Evelyn Nieves

"Educators Protest Limits on Multicultural Mandate," by Paula Ressler (see appendix)

"Gay Rights in California," *New York Times* editorial

Factfile: Hetrick-Martin Institute

"Youth Bring Gay Rights Movement to School," by Lamba Legal Defense and Education Fund (see appendix)

"Rainbow Over: Watered-Down Version of Teachers Guide to Make Rounds," by Liz Willen

Materials

Large newsprint paper

Markers

Summary

In this drama, a school community comes together to assume social responsibility for changing homophobic and racist attitudes and preventing hate crimes.
The new principal of a high school—the former principal recently retired—calls teachers and other staff members together to discuss the related problems of homophobia and racism in the school and to figure out what can be done to change the climate of hatred and fear that seems to pervade the community. The principal calls the meeting after an article appears in the *New York Times* about a school nearby. In this mostly white, middle-class community, Asian American, African American, and lesbian and gay students have been targets of violence and harassment. For example, a Chinese American student was beaten by teens and told to go back to China; white students performed a skit that stereotyped African Americans; and swastikas, other hate graffiti, and racial epithets have become common features of sports events.

What precipitated the article in the *Times* was a recent violent attack on a gay student who, after he announced he was starting a gay/straight alliance, a group in which gay and straight students could talk freely about issues concerning sexual orientation, was ambushed and beaten, and had the word *FAG* scratched on his stomach and arms. The principal of the high school was fired because he did not put a stop to the harassment, which had been building.

The new principal says that he is worried about what might happen at Pleasantville, a community very much like the one described in the *Times,* and has invited a queer student who has been harrassed, as well as a queer teacher and a parent to the meeting to help the community better understand the potential for violence at Pleasantville High. The guests also link racism and homophobia, showing how the two interconnected prejudices have created a climate of fear and hatred that makes it impossible for many people in the community to learn and thrive.

After hearing from the guests and asking questions to better understand their concerns, participants now step into roles as sexual minority students and as parents in the community. In small groups they explore the concerns and questions of each of these groups in the community.

Building on these concerns and questions, they all step back into role as teachers who develop action plans to address issues of safety, curriculum, and the need for overall structural reform.

Welcome Teachers to Meeting

The primary facilitation of this drama is carried out by the workshop leader in role as principal. If he is the sole facilitator, he will also be stepping into role as the guest student, teacher, and parent.

The drama begins when the principal welcomes the staff to the faculty meeting. He hands out the article from the *New York Times* (Nieves 1999) about a gay student who was attacked and the history of racist and homophobic incidents in a nearby community and asks everyone to read it. The principal also mentions the suit brought by Jamie Nabozny, a high school student who sued his school district for almost $1 million and won because it failed to protect him from antigay harassment that administrators knew was occurring.

Objectives

Beginning the drama with the welcome places the participants into role immediately. Discussing the article about the San Marin High School attack and information about Jamie Nabozny's lawsuit early on in the drama introduces important content information about the particular types of violence directed against LGBT people; the ways in which racism and homophobia are often linked; and successful efforts to address the discrimination faced by sexual and gender minorities.

Student Addresses Teachers

To help the staff better understand the issues, the principal has invited several people in the school community to talk about their concerns, both people of color and white people. The first speaker is a lesbian, gay, bisexual, transgendered, transsexual, or intersexual student who has been harassed and who is reluctant to speak.

The student should begin her narrative to the teachers with a statement about not wanting to be there and feeling too uncomfortable or angry to talk about what has happened. The participants in role as teachers must draw her out. When the student finally says something, she speaks about the tension in school with peers and the fact that teachers and administrators will not do anything about the incidents of harassment that have been occurring. The student is thinking of dropping out of school.

Facilitators in the role of the student have tended to begin their narratives with the following types of comments: "The principal asked me to come here, but I don't see why it should make any difference." "The only thing that will make things better is to get out of this place." "This is the second high school I have tried and the same thing keeps happening."

Objectives

This is an opportunity for participants to learn more about the types of difficulties that sexual minority students experience in school. To prepare for this role the facilitator might want to read student accounts of the pressures they experience, or the work of professionals who work closely with these students (Gordon 1983; Harbeck 1992; Herdt 1989; Heron 1995; Hetrick-Martin Institute 1992; Hunter 1990; Owens 1998; Remafedi 1994; Romesburg 1996; Savin-Williams 1992; Sears 1991; Telljohann et al. 1995; Unks 1995; Uribe & Harbeck 1992). The *New York Times* article handed out earlier will also be useful.

The teachers ask questions and offer support to draw the story out of the student, who is reluctant to talk. Participants go more deeply into their role as teachers as they try to help a reluctant and frightened student express her feelings and articulate her needs. In the process they also learn more than they knew about the harassment and danger facing sexual minority youth and experience the deep pain many such youth suffer in schools.

Lesbian Teacher Addresses Colleagues

Next the principal introduces one of the teachers, who explains that it is not only students who are having difficulties, but teachers too. (Note that this character could be gay, bisexual, transgendered, transsexual, or intersexual.) She worries that even addressing her colleagues at this meeting could be the beginning of the end of her teaching career. She talks about life as a lesbian teacher having to hide who she is and being frustrated and burned out because she cannot help her students. What brought her to the teaching profession was the fact that she cared, and after a few years in the system she is finding out that she cannot help the students who are most in need.

Facilitators in role as the teacher have made comments similar to the following: "If I could just reach out to the kids and tell them it is OK to be gay or lesbian, I would. But I was afraid I'd be fired. I walk into the cafeteria and every other word is 'faggot' and 'dyke,' even in the teachers' lunchroom. Teachers might use more polite words, but the prejudice is there." A Japanese American teacher in this role talked about the difficulty of coming from a very traditional background and not having the support of her family as a lesbian.

The teacher then goes on to say that she is sick of not being able to be fully herself and to reach out to students who need her. She lets her colleagues know that she is even considering giving up teaching. One such role-player said, "I'll probably earn more money as a tax consultant, anyhow."

Objectives

Again, this is a way to introduce more content knowledge into the drama about the needs of lesbian and gay teachers. Several books and studies would be useful background reading for the facilitator in this role (Epstein 1994; Griffin 1992; Harbeck 1992; Jennings 1994; Khayatt 1992; Parmeter & Reti 1988; Lipkin 1999; Sears 1992; Telljohann et al. 1995; Walling 1996; Woog 1995). The teacher also increases the dramatic tension in the drama by talking about the lack of support she feels from her colleagues. This will be discomforting for some of the participants in the same way that the student's story will make them feel uncomfortable. This tension also adds to the content knowledge of the drama. In order to incorporate new knowledge that leads to change, participants will first need to feel some emotional discomfort about having to assume responsibility for doing something about bias in the school, and then feel compelled to act upon those feelings.

Parent Speaks

The parent is upset about the new directions the school seems to be going in. He believes that it is important to uphold the values of the community and is concerned about someone new coming in and upsetting everyone. He is not sure that the school or school administrators should assume responsibility for the recent violence or that things are as bad as people are making it seem at this school. He also expresses the fears of some of the more vocal people in the PTA about the school promoting a gay curriculum or gay agenda.

"If Mr. Right were still principal, we wouldn't be having meetings like this. He knows it's only a few troublemakers causing all the problems. Besides, these students with piercing and tattoos and things like that are bringing it all on themselves. This used to be a peaceful community, then people started moving in who were so different. They don't care about their children like we do; they just let them run wild and do immoral things. What do you expect?"

Objectives

Facilitators can learn more about parent responses to antihomophobia education through newspaper articles, anthologies about sexual minority youth and families, and information published by Parents and Friends of Lesbians and Gays (PFLAG) (see Bozzett & Sussman 1990; Ryan & Futterman 1999; Woodman 1992). It is important to learn more about which parental fears and concerns are real and which are not, and which parents support making schools more welcoming for lesbian and gay youth and their families, which do not, and why. One of the strongest fears of preservice and new teachers is working with parents who are homophobic.

From the standpoint of the drama, the parent adds another dimension and point of view and more potential for increasing conflict as well as resolving it.

Teachers Step into Role as Students, Teachers, and Parents

After hearing from the three speakers, the facilitator asks the participants to break into four groups—students who are part of the Gay/Straight Alliance, another group of students who do not participate in the group, gay and straight teachers, and parents. Each group is asked to list what they know about homophobia and racism in the school and community, based upon the guest speakers' presentations and what they can add from their own experience, and then create a chart of questions and concerns about the current situation. The groups are encouraged to present as many different points of view as possible as members of the groups they represent. Each group then shares and discusses their list of questions and concerns with the rest of the participants.

Objectives

This is an opportunity for the groups to consolidate the information they have gleaned about different groups in the community. Dramatically, stepping into role as people who are directly affected by homophobia and racism is an important part of the work, through which people can bring their own concerns to the foreground in the role of someone else. This often allows people to express feelings and ideas they would not otherwise express and to experience the way other people perceive their feelings and ideas.

Teachers Address Safety, Curriculum, and Reform

The facilitator then asks the participants to all step back into roles as teachers and staff in the school and divide themselves into three groups to develop action plans that address issues of safety, curriculum, and structural reform. To clarify what is meant by structural reform, the facilitator passes out an editorial from the *New York Times* (1999) that talks about laws in California, Massachusetts, and Connecticut that prohibit discrimination based on sexual orientation. Each group develops an action plan to counteract and reduce homophobia and racism and is designed to make the school community a safer and more supportive environment for all students and staff.

Objectives

The purpose of this portion of the drama is to help empower participants to do something about homophobia and racism, two frightening and overwhelming topics for students and teachers. Even when no policies are in place to prevent teachers from talking about issues related to sexual identity, many teachers will assume that they will be fired for even answering student questions related to sexuality and gender identity. It is important to distinguish between when the threat is real, which it often is, and when it is not.

Giving participants the opportunity to creatively brainstorm and develop an action plan allows them to synthesize what they are learning with what they already know and empowers them to solve problems.

Guests Give Feedback to Teachers

After groups present their action plans, the facilitators in role as invited guests respond. They respond generally to the work the teachers have done, as well as specifically to the action plans they have developed. It is important for the guests to respond honestly and critically, as well as to be supportive of the participants' efforts.

Objectives

Guests responding to what participants are learning and demonstrating increases the perceived value of the work to the participants. Responding to specific plans developed by the participants also helps concretize their work and give it a place in the real world. Giving supportive but critical suggestions also helps push participants' thinking further.

Reflection

Everyone steps out of role to reflect on the drama as well as on how to build upon and implement action plans they began in the workshop. The objective here is to help participants make the mental transition from the hypothetical to the real as they think about how to put their plans into action in their own communities.

4

Socially Critical Drama Approaches

E arlier parts of this book discuss drama strategies in which the teacher is either in role or is tightly controlling important moments of the dramatic experience. The drama work in this chapter uses more of what Australian drama educator Edward Errington (1992) calls a critical drama approach. In this work the role of teacher is decentered and distancing techniques are used to create more emotional detachment and opportunities for critical reflection.

One of the earliest proponents of this approach was the German Marxist playwright and director Bertolt Brecht (Ewen 1967; Willett 1964). Brecht used techniques such as narration, titles, and characterizations that were larger than life to represent the forces of good and evil in the world, keeping the emotional response of his audience to a minimum, supposedly to allow more possibilities for critical thought.

This approach emphasizes bringing the student's life into the center of the classroom to help empower students to take charge of their lives, their learning, and their communities. Centered on questions posed by students rather than problems posed by teachers, it focuses on the relationship of the student to society and connects social change and activism to the curriculum.

The approach also demonstrates the curricular concept that less is more. It shows how exploring a topic in depth as opposed to covering a variety of topics superficially helps students develop their thinking and reasoning skills. It also emphasizes that giving students the opportunities to work out some of their social and emotional difficulties in the exploration of one topic may be more beneficial than superficial coverage of myriad topics in the curriculum. Working this way is about empowering students to

75

become engaged learners, critical thinkers, and agents for important social change.

This chapter describes three techniques that can facilitate a socially critical approach to drama. In each, the students work with a question they have about sexual orientation and gender identity, develop a scenario, enact it, and reflect upon it in terms of meaning and dramatic impact as well as implications for further learning and social action.

In preparation, students will read a book or an article, view a video, or experience a presentation about sexual orientation and gender diversity. Then they will write and discuss what they have learned from the texts. Next they break into small groups and brainstorm a list of questions or concerns that they would like to pursue further.

Tableaux

One useful technique that may facilitate the process of exploring problems related to sexual orientation and gender identity is *tableaux*, or frozen images. The tableau is a popular and versatile drama technique that is widely used by drama-in-education practitioners because tableaux provide manageable building blocks in the creative and intellectual process. These images are relatively easy to devise and can serve as scaffolding for the eventual preparation of fully enacted scenes. These human sculptures also help students distill the essence of a problem more easily by encouraging them to focus on important details involved in a dramatic experience, details they might ignore if they went directly into creating a full enactment of a dramatic moment.

Because the discussion, creation, rehearsal, and reflection that are part of the tableau process take time, the activity is designed to last for at least five sessions. In the first session, the class discusses the texts, breaks into groups, and brainstorms questions and concerns, such as the following: How do you come out to family members? How do you protect yourself from violence? How do you invite a friend home who doesn't know your mothers are lesbians? How do you present a poem that people would understand better if they realized the poet were gay? And so forth.

In the next session, each group will think of a key moment when a problem related to their question or concern has reached a crisis point: coming out to your parents; being attacked by a homophobic person in your karate class; your friend noticing your mothers' books about lesbians; students not understanding a Langston Hughes poem that has a homoerotic subtext. After having identified that moment, the group represents it in a tableau.

During the third session, the groups present their images to the others, receive feedback about the clarity and strength of the images, and revise the images, taking the feedback from others into consideration. The groups present the revised images and then create two more images: one that represents something that led up to that critical moment and another representing what may have happened afterward. This time, group members each add a word or phrase to each image they create.

In the fourth session the groups present their tableaux and receive feedback. They spend the rest of the session revising and rehearsing their new sequence of images. By this time, some of the groups may prefer to enact a scene more fully, with their three tableaux providing the foundation for beginning, middle, and end.

Students present their final work on the fifth day, rehearsing, performing, and reflecting on the process of creating their work. At this time, they also think about what else they need to know about the particular topic they have been investigating. Is there something more they would like to read or someone they would like to speak with in order to learn more?

Here is a student's written description of the tableaux performed in one session:

> Picture this: A Black student is on a basketball court and instead of watching him play, all his friends turn their backs on him. Picture this: one student harasses another student because he is gay. The student goes to a teacher for help and the teacher doesn't know what to do. Picture this: One student lying on the floor as if dead. Six other students stand in a semicircle around his head. Picture this: A young man asks a young woman to marry him. She says she can't because she has a girlfriend whom she loves more.

The most significant thing that this class came away with was a sense of getting close to issues they had never been in touch with before. One student explained: "Being close made me more sympathetic. When it doesn't directly relate to you it's hard. When the circumstances touch the emotions, it has a heavier meaning." Another student in the class at the end said, "God, I'd never thought of that before, that there are probably at least one to four gay people in each class."

Enacting and Reflecting on Personal Experiences

Australian drama educator Edward Errington (1992) outlines a highly accessible approach to creating socially critical drama. It involves taking a story through many stages of revision and rehearsal in order to delve deeply into meaning.

To begin the process, a group of five or six people first individually jot down an experience they have had or can imagine in relation to sexual orientation. They then recount their stories to one another and choose one to enact. Group members then ask questions to further clarify the experience, who the people involved were, where it took place, and what was really going on. This process takes at least one session.

Either the original storyteller directs or the group chooses someone else to be a director of the enactment. Everyone chooses roles. Everyone in the group needs to play a role, even if it's an inanimate object important to the story. Even the director must play a role in the story. Developing and rehearsing the scene takes at least one session.

Through improvisation, the group enacts the story, staying as close to the original version as possible. After the enactment the audience asks questions for the purpose of fully revealing the underlying meaning and significance of the story. The larger group will also make suggestions for the group to rework the story by asking questions about how time might have influenced the situation: What might have occurred beforehand that led to this story? What might occur in the future as a consequence? The facilitator asks the audience to invent a different ending, beginning, new characters, attitudes, cultures, settings. Imagination is encouraged to run free, often moving the story from realism to abstraction and symbolism. Depending on how many groups are involved, this part of the process can take one or more sessions.

The group then goes back to revise their story based upon discussion and other new insights. At this point, the teacher may suggest some reading or research that might help the group situate the story in a broader social context. Eventually the group rehearses and performs the revised piece for the whole group. Depending on the sophistication sought in the final version, the revision and performance process could take two or more sessions.

Once each group has completed the process, members write about and discuss what they have learned about their original scenario related to sexual orientation. They talk about what changed for them since the initial telling; how the enacting, questioning, rethinking, and revising process affected them; and how the activity transformed the knowledge they began with as well as themselves.

Forum Theatre

Brazilian theater artist and social activist Augusto Boal popularized many of Brecht's theater techniques in his work *Theatre of the Oppressed* (1974/1985) as well as Paolo Freire's educational ideas as propounded in his book *Pedagogy of the Oppressed* (1970/1993). Paralleling Freire, Boal's Theatre of the Oppressed (TO) calls for the democratization of education and the relationship between teacher and student as the foundation of social transformation. Boal's Forum Theatre, one form of TO, is a cross between political theater and social action. It starts with a social problem and invites audience members to explore various ways of solving that problem, breaking down the distinction between audience and actor. Members of the public replace the protagonist at a critical point in a drama and each enacts a different solution to the protagonist's problem. "So the seed of forum was to not give solutions, to not incite people. Let them express their own solutions" (Schutzman & Cohen-Cruz 1994, 23).

What is important about Forum Theatre is that people can pose their own problems and collectively try out a variety of solutions to each one. Participants in Forum Theatre are known as "spect-actors."* They are neither spectators nor actors, but audience members who are also participants in the drama. The idea of a forum is to give participants a safe environment in which to explore the social/political conflicts in their lives, find alternative ways to solve these problems, and eventually empower themselves to take action in their actual lives to end their own oppression.

Most Forum Theatre companies are composed of professional actors who invite audience members to join them in the process of problem solving by replacing the protagonist. In a traditional forum, actors work with a problem that is interpreted as a social conflict between someone who is oppressed and someone who is oppressing. They enact this conflict up to a turning point.

With the assistance of someone whom Boal calls the "Joker," a member of the audience will either replace the protagonist and continue the drama to take it to a point of resolution or replace the protagonist at an earlier point in the drama and then carry the conflict to another resolution. The Joker is the facilitator, who helps bridge the gap between actor and audience and the personal and the political, spells out the rules of the forum, and keeps the audience involved in the critical decision-making and problem-solving processes. Other members of the audience are continually invited to replace the protagonist and come up with different solutions to the problem. In addition to giving audience members opportunities to explore different ways to solve problems and break down the barriers between performer and audience, Forum Theatre and other forms of Theatre of the Oppressed also bridge a gap that exists between theater as performance and theater or drama for education and social change.

I adapt traditional Forum Theatre methods to meet my own needs as an educator. Because I do not do my educational work with professional actors but mainly with teachers and students in classrooms, my primary interest in Forum Theatre is the way it gives voice to multiple points of view and helps people explore difficult social issues creatively and collectively. It does

---

* Schutzman and Cohen-Cruz define Augusto Boal's concept of spect-actors as "engaged participants rehearsing strategies for personal and social change" (1994, 1). Through the spect-actor Boal breaks down the barrier between actor and audience, transforming the spectator from passive observer to active participant in the action (Boal 1992, xxiv).

this by deconstructing the binaries of actor and audience, theater and life. Forum methods create opportunities for critical reflection as well as empathic understanding. This often leads participants to change their consciousnesses while rehearsing new roles for themselves as activists in the real world.

In a classroom, I usually begin Forum Theatre work by asking participants to work in small groups to brainstorm and then explore a problem that concerns them or an aspect of a problem we are exploring together. This process can be facilitated as for the tableaux, creating first the moment of highest tension, then what led up to it, and finally what followed. I instruct the groups to develop a scenario and bring the problem to a point of crisis or conflict, enact it up until this moment, and then give other participants from other groups a chance to step into any of the roles the group created to try a different approach.

This does not exclude the possibility of people adding characters and roles to the drama, or stepping into what can be perceived as other than protagonist roles. Unlike Boal, I do not limit the choice of roles participants in a forum can play. Sometimes they take on the roles of people oppressed in the drama, sometimes the roles of oppressors. More often than not, I find these roles intertwine. It has been my experience that most situations that arise in educational settings are more complex than the binaries of protagonist and antagonist or oppressor and oppressed allow. A gay basher may be oppressed in other ways. A mother who cannot accept a child's queer identity is also struggling with her oppression as the parent of a sexual minority. In a drama about queer issues, the lines between oppressor and oppressed become blurred as in real life.

Pam Schweitzer describes how she too modifies Forum Theatre in her work in Age Exchange, a theater company working with the memories and current concerns of people between the ages of sixty-two and seventy-five in London. She said that she finds the model of oppressor versus oppressed, antagonist versus protagonist, inadequate for her needs.

> Where the oppression lies is often difficult to pinpoint in these situations; the power games we are showing are often so subtle that the perpetrators are not even aware of a conflict. Also, the roles of protagonist and antagonist are a shifting affair, and a fluid use of the Boal technique is required to maximize the impact of the audience's insights; that is, by modifying the forum convention of replacing only one oppressed protagonist in each scene, the conditions of oppression were more thoroughly unveiled. (Schutzman & Cohen-Cruz 1994, 80)

Students' initial enactment of a forum scenario is often superficial and sparse in detail. But the complexity of the initial conflict increases through continued reenactment and revision by others. This type of dramatic exploration often uncovers deep layers of meaning for participants, which inevitably leads to further discussion, research, writing, and sometimes, social action. I have found that students who participate in dramas of this sort come to understand issues from a variety of perspectives and points of view that may not have been available to them before.

The lines between oppressor and oppressed became very blurred in three forums created by students in a course I taught on lesbian and gay issues in classrooms. Each forum addressed a different aspect of working with queer issues in education as well as different challenges in terms of role-playing.

The first forum created by my students was a virtual classroom in which the topic of "What Is a Lesbian?" became the focus of the curriculum. The presenters of this forum stepped into multiple roles that lasted no more than a minute. The same people played roles of oppressor and oppressed, sometimes one right after the other, often blurring distinctions. For example, one female student, in role as a homophobic young man, defined lesbians as women who wore hiking boots and had hairy legs, the next minute she described them as women–loving women, and the next minute she stepped into role as a bisexual woman.

In another forum in this class, it was not clear who was more oppressed—a gay student who could not come out; his mother, who could not accept who her son was; or his teacher, who was gay but closeted and could not directly intervene to support his student. Participants in this forum played their roles more deeply and less stereotypically than those in the first forum. But they had difficulty moving the action forward to resolution because the closet became such an overpowering and constricting place for all.

Forum Theatres do not necessarily lead to resolution or answers to problems. They're more likely to lead to a fuller understanding of the problem and a desire to change social structures the participants may have encountered as frustrations during the forum. Forum Theatre should not be seen as a self-contained activity. This work needs follow-up, preferably through planning and implementing some social action. For example, the students in my class followed up their forum work with action research plans. Two students worked on curriculum projects to address a curriculum problem raised in a forum. Others made plans as to how they would come out as lesbians and gays in their workplaces. Two others focused on religious questions that had overwhelmed the characters they portrayed during the forums. One person planned to start a discussion group that would address the problems of sexual minority youth in her church, and the other rededicated himself to forming a new religious group that would accept sexual minorities, a project he had conceived several years ago.

Afterword

y own drama practice is inclusive of all the strategies, theories, and ideas included in this book. But no matter what strategy I am using at any particular time, my goals are always the same: to help make a difference in my students' lives. To accomplish this, I am engaged in trying to make schools safer for everyone, including les/bi/gay/trans people and their families. Engaging in this process is also about transforming schools from transmission-based, one-size-fits-all, teacher-centered environments into learner-centered, multicultural, feminist, and democratic environments in which everyone is valued and appreciated, and in which we can examine our fears and resistances to new knowledge instead of avoiding anything that challenges the status quo. The emphasis is on posing problems in multiple ways along with creative problem solving. Doing this work through drama emphasizes the importance of student voices and the need to create democratic classrooms in which personal experience can also be shared and challenged, where differences can be acknowledged, and emotions valued along with intellect. This work brings marginalized and previously suppressed voices to the center of inquiry, including those shaped by gender, sexuality, race, ethnicity, social class, and ability, for the purpose of changing consciousness and taking action to create a more just and equitable society (Fisher 1987; Schutzman & Cohen-Cruz 1994).

In the process of putting together this book and reflecting on the work I have done over the years, I have come to the conclusion that I have learned just as much from the participants I have worked with through educational drama as they have learned from me. I see my prime contribution to the learning experience as giving people an opportunity to participate in a difficult conversation that they would not have had otherwise. As a result of their participation, people gain the opportunity to reflect on their own thinking about identity, begin to see identities that seemed normative as social constructs, and can begin to question their previous assumptions in the light of what they are learning that is new. What transpires when people are given such opportunities continually fascinates and inspires me.

I want to thank everyone who has participated in the drama work I have developed and facilitated for offering suggestions about how to make my work more effective. Based on participants' suggestions, I have tried to integrate more video, music, and art into the work as a way to draw on people's many strengths, intelligences, and vehicles for learning. Participants in these workshops have responded very well to linking issues of racism and homophobia while acknowledging their differences. I continually try to make these connections more explicit in my work. In addition, I have added bibliographic resources and articles about specific issues that workshop participants have signaled as important. I have also listened to the voices that have asked me to spend more time on discussion and reflection, even when there is so little time and space available in which to step into role.

I have also learned to welcome workshop participants' negative feedback along with their positive comments. The honesty with which people have responded to working with LGBT issues through drama has been tremendously moving. People have shared their own stories, confusions, excitement, even anger. To me, this is the most hopeful sign that change is indeed possible. Often, expressing one's feelings about an issue, even when the feelings are negative, is the first step necessary in setting the stage for transformation. I do not think that homophobia is any more inevitable than racism or anti-Semitism. But it will take enormous efforts, sometimes in very small increments, in order to make a dent in people's deeply held prejudices. It will also take many people doing whatever they can wherever they can, at the same time that we struggle for opportunities to do deeper and more extensive work.

The work I have done confirms what progressive educators have said for decades, that information alone does not change hearts and minds. People also need a chance to explore feelings and ideas in a nonjudgmental atmosphere, time to test out their ideas with others and revise their thinking, time to create and re-create relationships and experiences, as well as time to investigate their individual questions and areas of concern. And, they need time to reflect on all these processes and experiences as well as opportunities to put new ideas into action.

It is my hope that the drama work suggested in these pages will inspire teachers to try out new ways of teaching and will help bring marginalized voices into the center of inquiry by opening up the conversation about sexual orientation and gender diversity in our schools. I am lucky to have been given many opportunities to do my work and to create opportunities where they didn't yet exist. Not everyone will enjoy similar possibilities. Nevertheless, I believe that whatever we can do in each of our particular circumstances to open up these important conversations will contribute to the creation of a more just and caring world, an environment that is healthier for everyone, where no one will be attacked for being who he is or loving whom she loves.

Appendices

Youth Bring Gay Rights Movement to School

David Buckel

Staff Attorney, Lambda Legal Defense and Education Fund
From the Fall 1999 *Lambda Update* newsletter

A recent study of lesbian and gay youth showed that the average age for young men to identify their sexual attractions as gay dropped from the year 1979, when it was around age 20, to 1998, when it was age *thirteen.* This study, conducted by Professor Ritch Savin-Williams at Cornell University, is more evidence that today, sexual orientation issues are smack dab in the middle of the nation's secondary schools—it is in grades seven through twelve where Lesbian/Gay/Bisexual/Transgender people are coming out in large numbers. But, as has always been the case in civil rights movements, when people first stand up proudly, bigotry lashes back most loudly. Many of us remember the news photos of African-American children, heads held high, walking to school while white people shouted and spit at them. Today LGBT students are trying to hold their heads up high, as they too are confronted with bigotry and abuse in public education settings.

The widespread nature and effects of that abuse are startling. Gay-identified students are the most likely victims of violence in school (according to a 1997 Minnesota Attorney General school safety report), five times more likely to skip school because they feel unsafe (Massachusetts Dept. of Education, 1995), seven times more likely to have been threatened/injured by a weapon at school (Vermont Dept. of Education, 1997), and four times more likely to attempt suicide than their peers (both Massachusetts and Vermont studies). In a study of gay-identified youth in 14 U.S. cities, 22% of males and 29% of females reported being physically hurt by another student in school, and 7% reported being hurt by a teacher. In a Gallup poll of American students age 13–17, the largest number said that gay students are the most vulnerable to harm from violent students, and that "hatred of gay people" is one of the most common topics voiced by violent students.

Many LGBT teens, who should be planning for a bright future, are instead having their hopes and dreams beaten out of them, emotionally and physically.

Lambda's precedent-setting *Nabozny* case has paved the way for significant improvements in the schools. The case's $900,000 price tag—set by the jury which held a Wisconsin school liable for failing to stop anti-gay abuse—led school districts to take the issue more seriously. Eight other lawsuits have now furthered *Nabozny*'s impact by using and expanding on its equal protection theories, often with Lambda's assistance.

For those many families who cannot go to court, perhaps because the parents and child have already endured too much pain to consider litigation, Lambda has identified an alternative beyond simply negotiating with the school: a Title IX complaint to the Office of Civil Rights (OCR) in the U.S. Department of Education. The OCR is not a court, and can only address bias tied in some way to sex discrimination, but it has the power to make a school safer. For example, the OCR may be able to address the bias of school officials responding to complaints of anti-gay abuse where girls are targeted for being "too masculine" or boys for being "too feminine" because this is sex stereotyping. Another common occurrence is when harassed boys get the official response that they should, unlike girls, take care of the harassment themselves through physical violence in order to learn how to be "real men."

Lambda paved the way for this alternate route in the *Wagner* case in Arkansas, which resulted in an overhaul of the Fayetteville Public School's sexual harassment policies, procedures, and trainings. That success has been replicated in Kentucky by a mother who complained under Title IX about the sexual harassment that her son suffered in school along with explicitly anti-gay harassment. In June 1999, President Clinton, in his Proclamation of Lesbian and Gay Pride Month, cited the work of the OCR as an example of the government working for the gay community.

We are also challenging the vocal minority of anti-gay parents who expect public schools to tailor curricula to individual prejudice. Working with the California Teacher's Association, Lambda obtained a cease-and-desist order against administrators who were granting parents' requests to remove their children from class because the teacher was gay, and we are now litigating a similar case. This work broadens our efforts on behalf of teachers and in support of schools' inclusive curricula, because the presence of gay people in classrooms and in textbooks is necessary to give LGBT youth positive role models.

Most exciting of all, students themselves are now organizing against harassment and violence, forming hundreds of Gay/Straight Alliances (also known as GSA's) all over the country, from Alaska to Nebraska, Arizona to Georgia. Schools' reactions have varied from a warm embrace of the students' initiative to threats to axe all non-curricular clubs to stop a GSA. Only Salt Lake City has been willing to terminate other clubs in order to block a GSA, and Lambda is lead counsel in a challenge to that drastic action. This summer, the

Manchester, New Hampshire school board grudgingly gave a GSA the green light, conceding it would lose a lawsuit enforcing the Equal Access Act, which requires federally funded schools to allow all non-curricular student groups equal access to school meeting rooms and resources.

Lambda has helped over 20 GSAs around the country to persuade school officials that their fears about such groups are unfounded. Many officials worried that allowing a GSA would "endorse" homosexuality, until we pointed out that the fear of "endorsement" does not extend to other non-curricular student groups like Bible Clubs, Young Democrats, and Young Republicans. We advise other officials who suggest that parental consent would be necessary for a student to participate in a GSA that, to be fair, the school would have to take on the burden of collecting parental consent forms from all groups. Some schools backed off entirely, one adopted our alternative suggestion that it send parents a list of clubs, instructing them to discuss at home which ones were appropriate for their children.

One of our plaintiffs in the Salt Lake City case reported a beneficial effect of all the publicity over her GSA. As the student harassers realized that the GSA members were a group, that many straight students were involved, and that they helped each other, some of the harassment stopped.

Lambda will continue working for youth in secondary schools by using legal tools to stop harassment, by supporting GSAs, by protecting gay teachers as role models, and by supporting schools with inclusive curricula, all to ensure that young people can believe in themselves, dream their dreams for the future, and always know that they are NOT alone.

PFLAG Fact Sheet

Parents, Families, and Friends of Lesbians and Gays (PFLAG), Bloomington–Normal, IL

Students At Risk[1]

Students who describe themselves as gay, lesbian, or bisexual and/or who have had same sex sexual contact reported being significantly more likely than their peers to face threats, attempt suicide and abuse drugs and alcohol. When compared to peers, this group was:

> ➢ 2-6 times more likely to have attempted suicide (and may account for 30% of all completed suicides.)[2]
> ➢ 5 times more likely to miss school because of feeling unsafe.
> ➢ Nearly 5 times more likely to have used cocaine.

Additionally, gay, lesbian and bisexual youth:
> ➢ Make up 20-40% of the homeless youth in urban areas.
> ➢ Have a much higher high school drop out rate (a recent study reported 28% of male teenagers self-described as gay or bisexual dropped out of high school because of verbal and physical abuse.

Reported Behaviors	GLB Students	Other Students
Was target of offensive comments or attacks Re: Sexual Orientation at school or on the way	34.4%*	6.3%
Was threatened/injured with a weapon at school in the past year	18.6%*	10.6%
Was injured a physical fight in the past year that required medical attention	14.9%*	5.1%
Skipped school in the past month because of feeling unsafe on route to or at school	20.1%*	4.5%
Feels unsafe or afraid at school some, most or all the time	20.9%*	11.9%
Smoked cigarettes in past thirty days	62.1%*	35.2%
Used cocaine in their life	31.0%*	6.8%
Has engaged in high risk drug use	35.8%*	22.5%
Was pregnant or had gotten someone pregnant (Percentage among sexually active students only)	31.6%*	11.8%
Has seriously considered suicide in past 12 months	34.4%*	16.7%
Has made suicide plan in past 12 months	31.1%*	15.7%
Has actually attempted suicide at least once in the past year	20.6%*	6.7%
Suicide attempt required Dr/Nurse intervention	9.4%*	2.2%

* Difference between Heterosexual and GLB Youth Significant at p<.01

---

[1] Data taken from the 1995 Massachusetts and Vermont Youth Risk Behavior Surveys, the 1995 Seattle Teen Health Risk Survey, and the 1999 Safe Schools Coalition of Washington publication
[2] Secretary's Task Force on Youth Suicide, U.S. Department of Health and Human Services

Gay/Straight Alliance Flier

Intersexual Drag Androgyny Woman KING Female TRANSGENDER Boy
Queer Homophobia Orientation Boy GENDER Femme Identity Butch Transsexual STRAIGHT .

GAY / STRAIGHT ALLIANCE GROUP

!EVERYONE IS WELCOME!

-THIS IS A GROUP WHERE YOU CAN ASK ALL THE QUESTIONS YOU'VE ALWAYS WANTED TO, BUT WERE AFRAID TO ASK ABOUT SEXUAL ORIENTATION AND GENDER IDENTITY!

-THIS IS A GROUP FOR LESBIAN, GAY, BISEXUAL, STRAIGHT, TRANSSEXUAL AND TRANSGENDERED STUDENTS WHO ARE QUESTIONING THEIR OWN GENDER AND SEXUAL IDENTITY.

-THIS IS A GROUP FOR PEOPLE WHO HAVE LGBT FRIENDS AND/OR RELATIVES.

MEETING: DATE:

                TIME:

                WHERE:

Queer Homophobia Orientation Boy Transsexual STRAIGHT Queen Gay Lesbian Male Bisexual
Drag Androgyny Woman KING Orientation Boy GENDER Femme Queer

Batty Boys in Babylon

Can Gay West Indians Survive the "Boom Bye Bye" Posses?

*Peter Noel with Robert Marriott**

"If a man is thinking of homosexuality, he's thinking of disease and wrong-doings, so God Almighty himself hates homosexuals. In Jamaica, if a homosexual is being found in the community, then we stone him to death."
—Shabba Ranks

"He that is without sin among you, let him cast the first stone."
—"God Almighty himself"

Eight years ago in the slums of Trench Town, Jamaica, a would-be murderer named Slicksta threw the first stone at Douche, a homosexual who loved to drag in *poom-poom* shorts and emulate the swagger of a rude batty woman.

"I stoned 'im. I beat 'im with sticks. I'm proud of it," Slicksta growls as he recalls the incident for a reporter and friends while browsing in Ethiopian Taste, a record shop on Nostrand Avenue.

The ambush occurred the day Slicksta was being initiated into a rudebwoy posse that roamed the alleyways of the island's shanty towns in search of the much reviled batty bwoys, as homosexuals are known. In these tin-can *dungles,* it's a mark of manhood to assault or even snuff a batty bwoy in cold blood.

The only real family dirt-poor Jamaican youths like Slicksta have is the Trench Town rudebwoys, descendants of "Johnny-Too-Bads" and "steppin' razors" of the '60s—the West Indian version of gangsta homeboys. But rude-bwoys are more than just "niggaz with attitude" running wild. Their posses are highly structured organizations, often led by a Don, the equivalent of a Mafia boss—and they can be as violent as L.A.'s Crips and Bloods. Their recruits, who signify with fustian patois, range from handsome waifs to snaggle-toothed "jungleness bad bwoys" and haunted *gunderleros* with their fingers on the trigger of a Mac-10, an Uzi, or a M-16.

Any rudebwoy wannabe would object to being called homophobic, insisting that he has no fear of homosexuals. He feels only rage. He would maim

93

or kill in order to achieve his objective: the capture of a batty bwoy to guarantee rank in the posse.

With the attack on Douche still vivid in his memory, Slicksta bites the lyrics of a Buju Banton song—"Man haffi de'd fi mek man live"—and savors Douche's agony with raw and uninhibited relish. "As I was beatin' 'im, I told 'im, 'Douche, y'u shouldn't be like dat.' Then I beat 'im. I stoned 'im. I beat 'im an' I stoned 'im. I beat 'im till 'im bawl, 'Murder!' I stoned 'im till 'im get away."

In Jamaica, hunting batty bwoys is as instinctive as the craving for *fry fish an' bammy*, a national dish. The mere sight of them can trigger the bedlam of a witch hunt. When the toaster (rapper) Hammer Mouth discovers two gay men in a garage—"hook up an' ah kiss like . . . meangy dog"—he hollers: "Run dem outa di yard." Murder them, advises another toaster, Bunny General. "Kill dem one by one. Murder dem till dem fi change dem plan."

According to local legend, the batty bwoy is a cruising vampire who sucks the blood of slum dwellers, called *suffarahs*. He will "chew y'u neck like ah Wrigley." He's a *duppy*—an evil ghost from Sodom and Gomorrah—not a human being.

In the deeply religious West Indian culture, many people still cling to Old World ethics. Their beliefs, morals, and suspicions are rooted in the canons of the Roman Catholic and Anglican churches, whose teachings on homosexuality are even more virulent in the former colonies than in Europe or America. In the West Indies, a priest who spots a confessed sodomite during the 40 days of Lent might single him out before the congregation and banish him with a sprinkle of holy water, or a recitation of the 14 stations of the cross. Many Jamaican Catholics believe they can atone for their sins by informing on gay or lesbian parishioners.

"Jamaicans are the most homophobic people in the Caribbean," asserts gay playwright Godfrey Sealy, who lives in Trinidad. "I've traveled to Jamaica and I know what it is like. They refuse to accept the fact that people are homosexual. Anyone found out to be so can be killed."

"Let's not stigmatize Jamaica," says Dr. Marco Mason, a Brooklyn-based Panamanian sociologist. "Homophobia permeates the region. It is something that is Trinidadian. It is something that is Barbadian. It is part of the culture of the Caribbean. Homosexuality is taboo."

But taboos feed obsessions and obsessions create curiosity. In the West Indies there are many ways to broach the forbidden. Dancehall—the new "hard-kicking, raw and wild" style of reggae—contains references to all manner of sexual prohibitions, including fellatio: "No ice-cream sound." As for cunnilingus: "How a man fi live inna 'oman hole like ah crab?" On the other hand, it's perfectly acceptable to "hear di y'ung gyal ah bawl when she get up tuh nine inch tall."

In Trinidad, the gay man is a *buller*, the lesbian a *zami queen* cursed with a *jumbie*, an evil spirit sent by an *obeah man*, the master of black magic. *Bullers* and *zami queens* can only be made straight—so the legend goes—when the *obeah man* himself is lured with bark, calabash, Julie mango, and angel hair and trapped in a rum bottle under a silk-cotton tree. The spirit of a *soucouyant*—usually an old woman who turns herself into a ball of fire and passes through a keyhole to suck one's blood—can also be beaten out of a *zami queen* with a *cocoyea broom*. But many West Indians—especially devout followers of the Rastafari faith—do not favor exorcism. They believe in the medieval punishments of stoning and burning. The batty bwoy, particularly, must be hunted down and killed.

So the stoning of Douche was "biblical," and killing him would have been the ultimate rite of passage for Slicksta, who was only 13 at the time. It's unlikely that Douche would report the attack for fear of further persecution by the police. Even well-known victims of gay bashing won't find justice in this Third World paradise. Between 1983 and 1988, many suspected homosexuals were stabbed or shot dead in Kingston. Among the more prominent victims were a physician, the principal of a prestigious boys school, a professor, an executive of the Caribbean Council of Churches, and a priest from Boston who was killed in his rectory. None of their assailants was convicted.

Buggery, however, is a felony in Jamaica, where police sometimes raid the homes of suspected sodomites. A deputy minister was arrested during one such raid last month, and charged with "aiding and abetting" a schoolteacher and his friend "found having sexual intercourse." The worst punishment of all was the embarrassment of seeing their names in the Kingston papers.

Since tourism is the island's main industry, gay visitors frolic without fear of the police. But the rudebwoy posses are not so tolerant of "blue-eyed devils." Heed Hammer Mouth's warning: "Bwoy y'u nuh fi test de murderer/Bwoy y'u nuh fi cross di border/Ah gwaan lick y'u doun ah groun'.'"

The situation in New York is not much better. The city's Human Rights Commission does not break down bias-crime statistics by ethnicity, so there's no way to measure the danger for gay West Indians on the streets of Babylon.

But Slicksta has emigrated to America. He's come to *Fareign* like an avenging angel on a winged horse breathing fire through its nose, eager to "chant doun" Babylon, the great Satan that breeds *duppies*, *jumbies*, and *soucouyants*. Whites need not fear his wrath; he hunts only West Indians. And in Brooklyn, Slicksta says, Douche is everywhere.

"I did it again on Empire and Bedford," he confesses, a bloodthirsty look in his eyes. "I saw a homo named Wilfred. I said, 'BOOyahka! BOOyahka! [the simulated echo of a gunshot, used as a salutation or death threat]. Batty bwoy, *divert*.' An' I stoned 'im. Dere is no rights fi batty bwoy. Ah lie, sah?"

"Y'u nah lie," answers his friend Passion, a 21-year-old Panamanian dancehall DJ who once played antigay reggae in Manhattan's Underground club, "jes tuh dis dem mama man an' batty bwoy." White gay men and their West Indian lovers bolted from the club. "Dey only have rights accordin' tuh Babylon society," says Passion, reaching for a popular dancehall 45.

"You ain't never heard of one great faggot prophet. Man, beat dem wid cable wire. Mih do it on mih block in Crown Heights aall di time."

"Papa San [a dancehall prophet] say, 'Put dem 'pon stick an' bu'n dem,'" a Trini Rasta scoffs, looking askance. "Jah kill ah whole city for dat."

Slicksta flashes a smile and waves the jacket cover of Buju Banton's *Mr. Mention* as if it were a flaming crucifix. "Look 'pon 'im 'ere," he beckons, admiring the coy but deadly profile of the 20-year-old *duppy conqueror* whose hit song, "Boom Bye Bye" advocates the execution of gay men.

Among rudebwoys in Babylon, Buju is a dancehall Don. He is the narcissistic "stamina daddy," a paramour who makes "gyal ben' down backways an' accept di peg." The worship of his *womb turner* and conquest of the *punani* (pussy) are the subjects of his burlesque boasts. Bashing the batty bwoy as he did in "Boom Bye Bye" is, as Freud put it, the "libidinal complement to the egoism . . . of self-preservation."

"What Buju is sayin' is dat dem [homosexuals] vex with *punani*," according to Slicksta. He insists that the reporter listen to the ultimate insult to the batty bwoy: "Can y'u please tell me," he toasts, "what 'appen with y'u an' di *punani*? Batty bwoy, why y'u sex-up Johnny? You're triple-freaky, sexin' man inna bottom aall night long. Kill di batty-fucker dem, one by one."

"How de fuck you could jes kill ah man?" I ask.

"Easy," Whiskey Bop Johnnie Walker, another Jamaican DJ, interrupts. "Batty bwoy haffi' de'd 'cause dem ah eat di bread from Sodom an' Gomorrah."

Combine this Old World intolerance with New World homeboy *kulcha*, and the batty bwoy in Babylon is placed in a precarious position. As Buju has instructed "all di New York crew," if any homosexual makes a pass at them, "is like, boom . . . inna batty bwoy 'ead" because "Brooklyn gyal" and "rudebwoy nuh promote no nasty man, dem haffi de'd."

Confessions of a Batty-Bwoy Hunter

Papa Bongo, a Grenadian ragamuffin with a nine-inch scar on his left cheek, checks his .380 magnum, kisses it, then tucks it into his waistband. He begins to tell the story of a *zami queen* he pistol-whipped in a Brooklyn dance hall for calling him "faggot" in the presence of his rudebwoys, but he stops in midsentence as a friend, with the cartridge of an M-1 rifle in one hand, lowers the volume on Natty B's "Puss," a homily on the sins of oral sex.

"Meh 'ave ah new name fi aall di bow-cat dem/When y'u see dem y'u fi point 'pon dem/'Cause dem ah puss, 'cause dem ah eat under frock/Dem ah puss, 'cause dem nah stop suck cock . . . . /Y'u come inna meh face with di hair inna y'u teeth/Y'u mouth, it smell like di renkin' meat."

"What is dat ah hearin'?" asks Bongo, whose homophobia is hair-trigger sensitive to prompts from anti-gay and lesbian toasts. "Lick it up," he orders his friend, who raises the volume. They chorus with Natty B: "Me an' Pimple . . . sight two bwoy 'ug up inna dance hall/So one ah dem 'ead inna di next one lap/So Pimple back he 'matie fi go lick two shot/Di bwoy dem say, 'Wait!' an' make big splash . . . "

The words are all too familiar to Papa Bongo. He wants to "massacre all ah dem. Ah whole heap ah posses should be huntin'—all dem Jamaicans, Trinidadians, Grenadians, Bajans, an' Guyanese batty bwoys an' lesbians go dead."

"So what happen tuh de *zami queen* who call yuh ah faggot?"

"Man, ah beat 'er mercilessly in she head," Bongo recalls. "Its ah word ah doh like. It leave ah lastin' stain on yuh."

A stain—like the stench of vomit and Old Oak Rum on the breath of his father, a stevedore who'd come home drunk, rip off his overalls, and beat Bongo and his mother. These days, the mere touch of a batty bwoy is enough to send Bongo running for his cutlass, which he used as a child to fend off his father. Did the *buller* who tried to touch Bongo at a fashion show in Flatbush have rum on his breath? This queer wearing Western chaps that exposed his batty—did he remind Bongo of his father?

"Ah wanted to kill him immediately," Bongo recalls. "Ah tell him not to touch me. But he touch me again, an' ah start to beat de batty bwoy like there was no tomorrow. If ah wasn't among so many West Indians who know meh, ah woulda shoot dis faggot in he head. 'Boom!' Like Buju say. 'Bye bye.'"

The next day, Bongo went to see his barber. "Ah was asking how long 'til he get tuh me when dis batty bwoy squeeze himself between us an' rub he cock against meh friend ass. People pull us off of him. From that moment on, ah declare war on dem. Anywhey ah see dem is big stone an' bullet."

Some nights, Bongo and his rudies will wander about, high on "Vat 19" rum and Guinness Stout, hunting batty bwoys. They stand outside West Indian dance halls in Flatbush, Crown Heights, or Jamaica, Queens, waiting to pounce. Right now, they plan to beat a bisexual man who is having an affair with one of their women. "She, ah eh go mention she name, jes like contaminated food now," Bongo says. "She have AIDS as far as we concern. We eh go kill 'er. She kill sheself ahready."

"All yuh go kill de man?" I ask Bongo, who once set a house on fire in Grenada when he and a group of friends discovered two homosexuals having sex. "If he dead from all de licks," Bongo snaps, "then dat's de way it shoulda happen."

Another target of the vigilantes is a posse of gay Jamaicans from Queens who drive around in expensive cars, wear huge gold necklaces, and pretend to be drug dealers. "All ah dem gay," Bongo claims. "Dey make dey money by sellin' theyself tuh rich white men. De rich men, dem is de 'oman, an' de batty bwoys is de studs."

One Friday, Bongo tried desperately to get through to *The Richard Bey Show* on Channel 9. The topic was gays in the military. "Ah wanted Richard Bey tuh know exactly what de gay soldiers did to de youts of Grenada," Bongo says angrily. He wanted to talk about the soldiers stationed in the rural district where he grew up. "De youts never see so much white men before. De white men had de guns. Dey had de power." Bongo believes the *tébé* (rumor) that some of the highest ranking officers were gay. "When de youts didn't succumb willingly, dey *man-rape* dem."

The Batty Bwoy Who Fought Back

It's dawn on Sunday. Most West Indians are ready to leave for early mass. But at The Shelter, a dank, cavernous underground in Tribeca, a loudmouthed Jamaican androgyne named Moi Renée is swinging his head to and fro, cocking his ass and twisting his hips with the grace of a Yoruban priestess possessed by an Orisha. He is wearing a body-fitted Emilio Pucci dress, black lace stockings held in place by garters, and Calvin Klein black suede pumps. His hair is festooned with colorful barrettes to imitate that West Indian *pickney* look.

"I am not a drag queen," he insists. And in fact, there's an edge of defiance in his apparel. He looks like a dance hall version of *Ole Mas* [a burlesque of master/slave couture] on *Jour Overt* morning [the start of Trinidad's carnival]. But his colors are pure Rasta: Red for the blood of Jamaican martyrs, black for his African ancestors, green for the fertile land and the hope of victory over oppression. And pink for his pride.

"I'd go back to Jamaica dressed like this," Renée dares. "I have a cult following."

But the singer, songwriter, dancer, actor, and comedian has not visited his homeland in more than 20 years. In Jamaica today, Moi Renée would be the perfect target of the Trench Town rudebwoys. If they ever ran into him on the streets of Kingston, they might "sen fi di matie an' di Uzi," as Buju Banton advises.

There was a time in Jamaica when Moi Renée, a shy, bedraggled *Dandy Shandy* playing nine-year-old, used to claw his brothers and sisters for calling him "'oman man" and "Mother Long Tongue." At the age of 11, he got into a fight with another boy. "He called me a batty man and we got into a fight. He ripped my shirt and stained it with his foot."

In 1971, Renée and his family emigrated to Philadelphia. He arrived in Babylon with the soiled shirt. The footprint of the batty-boy basher still haunted him. It came alive, kicking and stomping him every time he asserted his gayness. But there was nothing Renée could do to suppress that part of him.

"My first crush was on a black kid in my junior high school class named Keith," he recalls. "I was in love with Keith. He was so beautiful." The makeup on his face begins to crack as he recalls how Keith died. He was shot to death by a relative who "didn't like what he was. It was the greatest loss of my life."

It seemed as if every "Yankee boy" wanted to leave a footprint on his gay ass. "While I was still in junior high school the most embarrassing situation of my entire life occurred. I was accosted by a group of black boys and ordered at knifepoint to have oral sex with one of them. Of course I did it with reservation. I didn't want anyone to know, but the boys told and it got out into the school, and I was the big tease that semester. They were calling me homo, gay boy, and 'Faggot, faggot, you come from Jamaica and you're a faggot.'"

The taunting followed him to high school. One day, he ran into Vernon, the boy he'd been forced to blow. He heard those hurtful words again, but this time he lunged at his tormentor, stabbing him with a pencil. Renée had learned something about how to deal with bully boys in Babylon. The words didn't hurt him anymore.

Renée's life would become a series of struggles with potential assassins. One night, he was on his way to Mommy's, a gay club in downtown Philly, when two men approached him, asked for a dime, and when he said he didn't have one, called him a "Jamaican pussy." One of them, a muscular fella, slammed Renée in the back of his head. "I looked at him very calmly and said, 'You stand right here and I will be right back,'" Renée recalls. He'd seen a pretzel cart with a pipe iron propping up the wheel. Renée wasn't going for a pencil this time. He grabbed the pipe iron and began to pummel the stranger who had come out of the darkness like a *duppy conqueror*. He faded back into the night, tossing his afro pick at Renée.

In 1979, Renee moved to New York, to get away from his tormentors and increase his options. Here, a rangy West Indian man in Doc Martens and a designer frock could have a career. Renée has been a towel boy at the Continental Baths, a window designer at B. Dalton, and lately a *chanteuse* with his own single, "Miss Honey." He continues to test the tolerance level of West Indian heterosexuals by swishing through Flatbush. "If I feel like walking with a switch or behaving openly effeminate I do it," he boasts. "There are laws on the books here that people in my position should not be discriminated against. I feel proud to go out and be myself."

Undercover Lovers

It's late at Gill's Paradise, a safe house in Crown Heights where batty bwoys gather on Tuesday nights. Gill's introduces itself in burgundy letters daubed against a floodlit yellow facade. On a wall of the building is a mural depicting a Rasta crouching and petting a tiger in the shade of a palm tree. Some say he's taming the Conquering Lion of Judah. The symbolism springs to life on the crowded dance floor as two men with dreadlocks hug each other and bounce to the bass line of Tiger's "Come Again."

Not an unlikely scene in New York except that these are children of the West Indies *stick on like ants* and batty-riding in the face of the dominant culture. Other young men in baseball caps and Polo gear kiss, grind, and *wine* (a rhythmic pelvic motion) to the "hard and stiff" toasts of Shabba Ranks. Banjy boys check and recheck each other out in the corners of the room, while in the center of the floor, a hip-swinging Indo-Guyanese flames on.

The beat changes and soca music booms from the sound system. Everybody is jumping up to Crazy's "Take ah Man," a controversial song that has become an anthem of the gay West Indian underground. Now, its chorus becomes a sing-along: "She say, 'If yuh cyar get ah wooman, take ah man.'"

But they've come to Gill's searching for more than a man—and more than just a place to *shake dey kangkalang* like *jagabats* (whores). Under cover of disco darkness, they can *ramagé* (posture). In this hole, a *mamapoule* can be a rudebwoy. Or he can make his oppressor look like a *blasted koonoomoonoo* (damn fool).

The DJ slips on Buju Banton's "Bogle"—"de wickedest dance from outa J-A,"—and the crowd is hyped. They contort their faces in a blowsy *pappyshow* (parody) of Shabba Ranks's funnel-nosed grimace and Buju's fatal attraction. Slouching and prancing like court jesters with a snap-queen attitude, they burlesque the peculiarities of the Bogle, as if this dance were invented by a gay *gundelero.*

"Fling y'u han' inna di air," Buju instructs, "then y'u rock an' y'u dip/Move tuh di drum an' mek y'u body kick/Step farwod an' come-up back quick."

"BOOyahka! BOOyahka!" the revelers shout back, their fingers extended in the shape of pistols, shooting up the night. "BOOyahka! BOOyahka!" But none of these batty bwoys "get up an' run,"—Buju's advice to gay men if they don't want to be shot. They're drawn to the rudebwoy *stylee:* to its power, its allure, its recklessness—its resistance to oppression. For them, the Bogle is not a show of aggression but of cultural connection despite rejection.

But the fantasy is short lived. One by one, these Ba'd Johns drop their "guns." All of a sudden, BOOyahka seems too real a threat. How can they make fun of such terror? How can they dance to the executioner's song?

At Gill's Paradise and other such clubs, gay and lesbian West Indians "may appear invisible because it is impossible to live safe and affirming lives," according to Colin Robinson, a Trini who is cochair of Gay Men of African Descent. "Many of us, like me, 'cross over' into the relative safety of the African American gay community where we become 'Black Gay Men' . . . We don't challenge our own communities and families. We laugh along with the *buller man* jokes [and] bite our lips at the hatred our mother casually displays at the dinner table for the people she doesn't know are us."

Desmond's mother never told such jokes at the dinner table. A traditional Guyanese mother would never discuss any aspect of sex with her children—not even with her Yankified 17-year-old son. But Desmond's stepfather, an Antiguan, felt no urge to suppress his disdain for *auntie-men*. He had his suspicions about Desmond's sexuality. One Saturday morning, he searched his stepson's dresser drawer and found some condoms. Desmond was shattered—his mother must not know. He told his stepfather that he'd bought the condoms because he was "bonin'" several hotties. The stepfather was not convinced.

A few minutes later, he interrupted a conversation between Desmond and his mother. "Me think you *pickney* ha' sum'n fu tell you," the stepfather snarled. For months, he'd been dogging the youth's every move. The badgering made Desmond's stomach wamble. He headed for the bathroom but the stepfather followed him and there he confronted Desmond again.

"Me find dis flyer inna you pocket," the stepfather growled. He produced a promo for The Men's Room with a photo of a naked man groping his dick. "Me min call dem an' dem tell me dat ah one big *auntie-man* place. Me tell dem, 'If you ever let a minor into your club again I would do whatever I have to do.'"

"What you talkin' 'bout?" asked Desmond, throwing his hands in the air. "Step off! Why you on ma jock?"

"*Tell* you muma," his stepfather demanded.

Desmond dallied in the bathroom for two hours before coming out to face her. "Is wha' goin' on?" she asked.

The stepfather interrupted: "Me think you *pickney* ah one big *auntie-man.*"

"Desmond, dis true?" she asked. Her son looked away. Something in him wanted her to know. "I ain't nevuh slept with no man before," he mumbled. "But I *do* find them attractive."

His mother was the only woman Desmond trusted. He would talk to her about everything else except this. But now she stared at him in disbelief. The silence between them was an embarrassment he had never imagined.

"You think you could change?" his mother whispered. "Becuz as long as yuh livin' under me roof yuh gon can do dat."

Had this scene unfolded in Guyana, Desmond's mother might have made immediate plans to drive the *obeah* from her son. But because they were living in Babylon, the youth was sent to a psychiatrist. Therapy, however, did not prompt the devil to depart. In fact, Desmond soon became engrossed in a relationship. "I was still in school and I was working part-time, but I would come home every morning at six. My stepfather was always on my case."

On the morning of his 18th birthday, Desmond came home late. His mother had waited up for him. She was dressed for church. "You gon can do dat an' live here," she said sadly.

Desmond reached for his teddy bear. "Guess what?" he blurted, glaring at his stepfather. "I'm outta here."

Few West Indian mothers ever find out about their gay sons and daughters. "No," says Mayaro, a 24-year-old Trini who is a regular at Gill's, "my family don't know. Dey would kick meh outa de house or try tuh beat meh straight."

Four months ago, however, Lopinot, another 21-year-old "middle-class Trini," bared his secret to his mother, a devout Catholic. "It was hard for her because of all the religious mythology around homosexuality in Trinidad. But I had to make my mother understand that Lopinot now is still the same Lopinot from before she knew I was gay. I had to make her understand that it was still me."

Moi Renée understands their pain. He mourned his first love, Keith, alone. He learned to fight the bashers on his own. Even though his family has always "known," they've never talked openly about his life, until Renée called up his brother Naphtali to wish him a happy birthday.

They had not spoken in years. Naphtali is a member of the Twelve Tribes of Israel, an offshoot of the Rastafari movement. The Twelve Tribes is built around reggae, the music of the King. Bob Marley was their "chief singer and player of instrument." The sect, known as the Uptown Rastas, embraces *di black petty-booshwah* who were afraid to go into the ghetto to join the Vintage Rastas. It has chapters in Babylon and even accepts whites as members. But no Twelve Triber who claims to "deal at a higher level of consciousness" would be caught dead accepting birthday greetings from a homosexual. Even from his own brother.

"I an' I nah want no happy birthday greetings from y'u," Renée recalls Naphtali telling him. "Y'u still into dat faggotism? If y'u still ah batty man, me nah want talk tuh y'u."

"That's my business," Renée choked. Under the anger, he kept thinking of his brother as a baby, and it made him want to sob. "When you were a child," he asked at last, "who do you think took care of you?"

The brother hung up.

In the West Indies, Twelve Tribers won't speak to their homosexual siblings. But here in Babylon, many devotees are rebelling against the strictures of their religion. Some have embraced gay friends and relatives. Others have discovered that they are gay.

Lost in Babylon

Yula seemed annoyed by the whinny of the iron horse as it chugged through the belly of the beast. But the petite woman who sat across from her was a momentary distraction. The sister, whom she'd later come to know as Winsome, was dressed in a flowing white cotton dress hemmed with red, green, and gold sashes. Her matted dreadlocks were wrapped in a coarse white hairnet that identified her as a member of the Twelve Tribes.

Yula was a rebel Rasta born in Babylon. She was dressed in blue jeans and a white T-shirt. Other Rastas, disapproving of such attire, would go out of their way to condemn her. "Sistren," they would snap, that would be a Biblical rebuke—"Get thee hence, Satan"—because Yula "look good but t'un bad." Her mannish swagger gave her away as a *bow-cat*—a woman who would *nyam any niggle* (eat pussy) and refuse to *bumflick 'pon ah dick*. Yula tore her eyes from Winsome, looked at the ads for decongestants and hemorrhoid remedies, and tried to make her mind go blank.

The two women avoided further eye contact until the train stopped at Astor Place. Yula raced up to the street. She was standing at the corner contemplating her next move when she felt a gentle tap on her right shoulder. She spun around and came face to face with the woman she'd been trying to dodge.

"Sistren," Winsome asked the stranger in her Jamaican accent, "evah 'ear 'bout Pandora Box?" Yula nodded, dumbfounded. "Could y'u tell I an' I 'ow tuh get there?"

"Why?" Yula asked gruffly.

"I an' I jes wah go there," Winsome squeaked. But she was looking for more than directions.

"Why ask me?"

"I an' I trust y'u 'cause di sistren is ah Dread."

"Do you know what kind of club this is?"

Winsome giggled, girlishly. "You asked the right person," Yula said. That seemed obvious to Winsome.

"You straight up Rasta?" Yula asked her. Winsome nodded yes.

Yula knew that there were gay Jah-fearing Rastas, but she had never met one. Suddenly, there were dozens of questions she wanted to ask—like how a lesbian could be a member of a sect that can justify the stoning of any member exposed as a homosexual. "Is jes sex," Winsome said abruptly. "I an' I 'ave sex any way I an' I feel like."

Winsome told Yula that she wanted to get married and have children but that she'd had sexual feelings for women all of her life. Yula had no such domestic fantasies: she'd always known what she was. "Femme in the streets, butch in the sheets," was her assessment of Winsome.

At Pandora's Box, Winsome's eyes opened wide, soaking in an ambience she could only have imagined back home. Here, she saw women of all shapes and sizes—most of them black—stalking and slinking or dancing on the tiny crowded floor. As Winsome stood against a wall, Yule made her move. "I just came up on her and I kissed her. And after that it was like, 'When am I going to see you again?' We made love the next weekend. She initiated the whole thing. It was her first full-blown homosexual encounter. I asked her, 'Are you sure you're telling me the truth?' She was very passionate. She knew what to do."

But Winsome confined her lust to their private encounters. "She told me that she was living with friends. Nobody should know. 'No, dey *can't* find out,' she kept saying. 'If dey find out, I an' I will be stoned.'"

"How do you deal with it?" she asked Winsome.

There was terror in her eyes: "Dey can't find out," she begged.

"Well, you have to come to terms with something," Yula insisted. "You exist and I exist. There have to be others like us, just like there are gay Christians and gay Jews. There *must* be gay Rastafarians. Let's make an Order."

In the end, the two women agreed to keep their relationship a secret. But something in their mien made even the smallest gesture of affection seem suspicious. One day, they were accosted by a dope-dealing Trini Rasta, who saw them walking hand in hand, like nuns. "He took one look at the both of us and he went off. He said, 'All yuh is ah disgrace tuh Rastafari. Cut off allyuh locks. Somebody should cut off allyuh locks.' I remember Winsome shouting back in patois, 'Y'u don't know I an' I relationship with Jah an' Selassie I! How can y'u judge I an' I?'"

No one had to judge Ambakaila. She'd condemned herself long ago. Drawn to women for all of her adult life, the *pickihead* tomboy struggled to bury those feelings beneath an even stronger attraction to men. But at the age of 30, Ambakaila met Marabella, her *doo-doo darlin'*, her first love. Their passionate affair knew no bounds, except to their *mauvais langue* neighbors in a close-knit fishing village in Trinidad. The constant finger-pointing and *shooshooin'* (tongue-wagging) destroyed their relationship, but not Ambakaila's feelings toward Marabella.

Ambakaila's *tabanca* (longing) for Marabella made her love-crazy. The only way to rid her heart of this *tololo*, or love-jones, was to get away. She fled to Babylon.

"Ah never wanted tuh live in America," Ambakaila recalls. But she'd decided that a *zami queen* did not deserve to be in Trinidad. She belonged in Babylon, with all the other sinners. "America was my way of punishin' mehself," she explains. "Boy, ah wanted to purge mehself, just bathe mehself in ashes. America was *my* sackcloth an' ashes."

Three years had passed since Ambakaila's arrival in Brooklyn, three years since her last encounter with Marabella. Ambakaila had begun to believe that God washed her conscience of all guilt. "Ah tell mehself, 'After three years of heterosexual love makin', I eh go have ah problem with dis again.' Ah went back tuh meh Baptist religion an' ah feel dat ah was like totally cured. Boy, it was three years ah jes prayers, praying real hard to God, tuh take dis t'ing away, whatever it was. Ah tell de Lord, 'Okay, ah go admit ah have ah attraction fuh women. Now take dat feelin' away nah because ah know dat it wrong. Please take it away.'"

But the feeling endured and it exploded the day Ambakaila met Sally Jean, a white woman who she insists is the spitting image of her lover Marabella. Sally Jean is openly gay and very active in her church. "She tell me dat she never felt closer tuh God. She say God talk tuh she an' tell she, 'It's all right. I accept you as you are. I am okay with you being a homosexual.'"

Ambakaila and Sally Jean became lovers, and slowly Babylon culture began to work its way with her. "She take meh aroun' tuh ah gay community center, gay bars, DT's Fat Cat: de landmarks. She tell me dat I should get tuh know other gay people an' dat ah was not alone in what ah goin' through."

Sally Jean introduced Ambakaila to Identity House, a gay counseling service. At first, she resisted attending the group sessions. "Ah wanted tuh talk tuh somebody. Meh own people, Trinidadians. But ah couldn't see mehself sharin' dis so-called secret wid dem. Ah jes make up meh mind one Friday evenin' an' ah went to ah group session. I get to find out dat it had plenty other people like me who have identity crisis. Dat is what I goin' through, an identity crisis. Ah lotta people come tuh de sessions an' find out dat all dey really had was ah homosexual experience. Ah lotta dem find out dat dey bi, some find out dat det gay, an' ah lotta dem find out dat dey straight. Dey find out 'bout dis thing in dem."

Ambakaila has attended three sessions. "De crisis more intense now if yuh ask me. Ah almost certain dat ah not gay, becuz ah does still lie down on meh bed an' fantasize 'bout takin' de biggest *totey* [dick] in town, even with all dis identity crisis ah goin' through. But then ah cyar remember evah havin' so strong ah feelin' fuh ah man as ah had fuh Marabella an' Sally Jean. So what does dat make meh?

"I tryin' tuh find answers tuh dis problem by handlin' it in ah vertical way: Me an' meh God. Up an' down. Ah try de horizontal method an' ah come tuh realize dat nobody in de Christian community would evah tell meh dat it's right an' ah could be gay an' godfearin'. An' nobody in de gay community would evah tell meh dat ah can't do both. Everybody would have dey strong arguments. Ah jes feel like ah in de center an' people from both sides pullin' meh, jes tearin' meh apart."

Could You Be Loved?

I was one Trini to whom Ambakaila could confide. After all, I was her co-pere, she my ma-comere. She was grim-faced and still wrestling with her maddening *tololo* the night she arrived unexpectedly at my Harlem apartment.

"Who dead?" I asked as Ambakaila brushed past me and dove onto the bed. I lay down beside her. "Girl, what happen? Yuh mudda dead? Yuh fadda dead?" She covered her head with pillows and began to bawl.

"Like somebody put *maljoe* on meh," she sputtered. "Everytime ah try to get on wid meh life de devil does come back like ah tick in meh *kakahole*."

Ambakaila was frightening me. "Yuh have AIDS?" I pressed.

"Nah," she replied abruptly. "What ah have more woss than AIDS."

"Cancer?"

"Stop fuckin' wid meh," she said angrily. "I jes ready fuh de *Labasse* [the city dump]."

I told Ambakaila that she needed a "bush bath or ah dip in de salt" to wash away the *maljoe*. But she'd already tried to cleanse her svelte body with blue soap, Florida water, and lavender.

"John John [my home name], all de *bacchanal* yuh use to hear 'bout me an' Marabella is de truth."

I had no inkling of what Ambakaila was talking about until she said it in plain English: "Marabella and I were lovers."

"And . . . ," I said, anticipating more details.

" . . . An' ah feelin' shame an' dutty. Ah want tuh bathe."

"Gyul, make de sign of de cross in yuh mouth."

"Yuh think yuh could still love meh like yuh did 10 minutes ago?"

"What kinda stupidness yuh askin' meh? Yuh soun' like ah scratch-up Bob Marley record: 'Could You Be Loved?' Cud yuh be-e-e-e luv? Ah still yuh *compeh*."

I had never seen Ambakaila cry. I'd never seen tears gush so violently from anybody's eyes. She handed me a ream of letters from Marabella, tearjerkers calculated to induce the most excruciating guilt and jealousy. I felt like tearing them up and siccing a *jumbie* on the author. In Trinidad, I would have *made a cook* and said a Novena for my friend. But here in Boo York, we fell asleep weeping in each other's arms.

The next morning, after she'd left, I phoned my brother Michael, who lives in "Crooklyn." I didn't know how to tell the *maco* (gossiper) that his suspicions about Ambakaila had been right all along. I could almost hear him lapsing into one of his *malkadies*, or fits, about my association with *bullers* and *zami queens*—"an' dat faggot newspaper" I work for.

"Here nah," I said to get his attention. "Ah bringin' Ambakaila tuh yuh party an' ah doh want yuh to play 'Boom Bye Bye.'"

"What she have tuh do wid Buju Banton?"

"Ent yuh say yuh ent want no homosexual in yuh house?"

There was a strained silence. For once in his life, the *maco* was witless. "Bring she," he huffed. "She come like famalee tuh me."

But Michael, who had introduced me to Bob Marley's message of "One Love," did not want me to bring any more of my gay friends. He didn't want them around his two impressionable boys.

Michael reminded me that, back in John John, the neighborhood in Port-of-Spain where we grew up, our grandmother had to protect four brothers from being hit on by a well-known homosexual called Mikey Mike. He told me I was the naive one because, while he and the other children would taunt Mikey Mike, I would hold lengthy talks with him.

"Mikey Mike nevah touch me," I told Michael.

"Becuz our grandmother woulda take night and make day for he ass if he *bull* we."

Michael agreed not to play "Boom Bye Bye" in Ambakaila's presence. "But ah go play it when she gone. Ah go play dah song jes fuh yuh skin."

Oh how I wanted to see the look on Michael's face when Ambakaila appeared. But she stood me up—and so did my daughter's favorite uncle, a fashion designer and Willi Smith devotee. So when Michael put his favorite record on, no one objected. My 11-year-old, Zanelia, who had heard this song on the radio, jumped up and chirped: "Boom bye bye inna batty bwoy 'ead. Rudebwoy nuh promote no nasty man dem haffi de'd."

She couldn't comprehend the meaning of the words, but she understood the look on my face. "This song is about your uncle," I explained. "It's about killing your uncle." There was an awkward silence as the tears streaked down her cheeks. Then she spoke: "Sorry, uncle. Bye bye, Buju."

Murder, He Wrote

The real "nightmare of the suffarahs" is not blood-sucking homosexuals. It is the *Gun t'ing* that has claimed so many Jamaican lives in recent years. "Gun t'ing," the toaster Hopeton Lindo cries, "is ah serious somethin'. Di youts dem nowadays not jokin'—especially when dem sniff dat white t'ing. Dey don't care who y'u are or where y'u from; di simplest t'ing is jes blam! Blam! Blam!"

Dancehall Dons such as Buju Banton lionize "gun murdarahs" and covet their notoriety. In "Man Fi De'd"—his warning to all informants who "chat out mih bizness"—Buju and his rudies are "no gun punka." In fact, he suggests that one informant "tell 'im famalee an' frien' fi prepare 'im Nine Night 'cause if mih buck 'im ah day, or if mih buck 'im ah night, mih can bet y'u I'll win—it nag go be ah pretty sight." In other words, "jes mek dem no we nah save no lead: gunshot fi buss-up inna informer 'ead."

Many dancehall enthusiasts, who "labba dem mouth like ah radio station," say Buju is just "woofin'"—or voicing the harsh realities of *jungleness*. But his obsession with the gun culture evokes more than idle threats. It's a synthesis of male posturing, sexual paranoia, and a political tradition that dates back to 1865, when a heavily armed Jamaican preacher, Paul Bogle, led the Morant Bay rebellion. That uprising helped end the tyranny of the British plantocracy.

Young rudies pattern their rebellious ways on Bogle's defiance. In fact, they've named their gun-posturing dance the Bogle after this freedom fighter. But this spirit of resistance became warped during the '80s, when Edward Seaga—a/k/a "CIAga"—came to power with an American-backed right-wing government. Armed posses suppressed dissent and the tradition of political violence became enmeshed with criminality. Bob Marley's admonition to Jamaican youth, never to forget Paul Bogle and "where you stand in the struggle" was forgotten as cavalier black-on-black violence exploded—in the ghettos and the music.

These "sound bwoys" of fury have put dancehall reggae, a traditional folk form, through virulent changes. "Dancehall is a different kind of phenomenon today," says Gladston Wilson, program director of the Jamaica Broadcasting Corporation. "It has drawn on some of the most vulgar elements in society in terms of talk, dress, attitude to each other, and it tends to speak in very violent language. Bob Marley talked about chasing 'those crazy baldheads outta town' because of injustice. People thought Marley was a revolutionary in a Marxist sense. He turned Haile Selassie's speech into a song called 'War.' But he wasn't saying you need to take up guns and shoot people."

Buju—who scoffs, "Mih nah laugh wid people, man. Mih kill people an' drink blood"—is too powerful an entertainer not to be taken seriously.

Last year, the toaster unraveled the moral fabric of a color-conscious Jamaican society with "Love Mih Brownin'," a song extolling the virtues of light-skinned women. Buju calls it "a likkle conflick," but Simon Buckland of *Reggae Report* writes that Buju "came under a lot of criticism [from] a number of recorded responses, the most notorious of which was Nardo Ranks's 'Them a Bleach,' a ditty . . . that directly lays the blame for black girls trying to bleach out their skin at the feet of Buju Banton."

The criticism forced Buju back into the studio to record "Love Black Woman." But the damage had already been done. "Times dere I was immature," he told Buckland. "Now I'm moving up, 'coming a man, so the vibes and material now is different, y'unnerstan'? If you listen the tracks from then and now, you'll recognize the big difference."

The "big difference" was that Buju Banton now suffered from batty-bwoy-on-the-brain, the dread of gays that compelled him—"a young man raised in the Carribbean"—to write "Boom Bye Bye." Last summer it was not uncommon to hear the lyrics being chanted like a mantra with intense cultural pride in Jamaica, the "small community" for whom he says the song was intended. Soon its notoriety spread to West Indian enclaves in Crown Heights, Flatbush, and Bedford-Stuyvesant. The song could not have emerged at a worse time: a new alliance was being forged between dancehall's gun-boasting rudebwoys and the gangsta strains of hiphop, which also expresses cultural pride through an almost playful ultraviolence.

"Boom Bye Bye" 's ominous message to gays was almost concealed behind a mask of banality, in which humor and violence intertwine: "Two man hitch up an' ah hug up an' ah lay down inna bed/hug up one another/an' ah feel up leg . . . /shoot dem now, come mek we shot dem."

By then Buju had left his small community. And by his own account, he "traveled the world" and saw the "*positive* [emphasis his] impact" that his music had in "diverse cities such as Tokyo, London, and New York." But Buju didn't fully understand the meaning of the words *diversity* and *tolerance* until the Gay & Lesbian Alliance Against Defamation (GLAAD) boldly defined them for him.

On October 21, GLAAD joined forces with Gay Men of African Descent (GMAD) to decode Buju Banton's bullet-riddled patois. The two groups embarked on a media campaign to have "Boom Bye Bye" removed from the playlists of radio stations WBLS and WRKS. Three days later, a front-page headline in the *New York Post* declared Buju's song "HATE MUSIC."

Buju, the rudebwoy with the "crocodile 'eart an' iguana stomach," says he meant no harm. "The antigay sentiment expressed in the lyric was, and continues to be, very much a part of the Caribbean culture," he reiterated. Buju's response has triggered a heated debate over whether homophobia—and even gay bashing—are imbedded in West Indian tradition, and if they are, whether artistes like Buju merely reflect the culture when they express contempt for homosexuality. (Buju has refused repeated requests for interviews from North American media: he was unavailable for comment to the *Voice*.)

Despite a ban on antigay dancehall by radio stations, many Jamaicans here and *backayard* insist these dancehall rudies remain true to the culture. Batty-bwoy hunters and gun murdarahs, they claim, are alter egos. They quote Shabba Ranks to shut you up: "I know mih roots an' culture/Murdarah! It is music mih charge fah/Murdarah!"

Dr. Luther Blake, a Jamaican-born political and educational consultant, who lives in Brooklyn, forsees a "change of attitude" toward homosexuals in the next generation of West Indians.

"They will eventually change," Blake asserts, "just as many things in the Caribbean have changed. Whoever thought 30 years ago there would be a black power movement in the Caribbean? That's happened. They may be 10 to 15 years behind this country, but eventually there will be an openly gay movement. You may end up seeing gay bars in certain places like Jamaica, a concept that seems completely radical now. When West Indians begin to see gay people as just people and not some kind of aberration then they'll learn to deal with them."

—P. N. & R. M.

*Some names and physical descriptions have been changed at the request of the subjects. The authors acknowledge: *The Rastafarians* by Leonard E. Barrett Sr.; *Creole Talk of Trinidad and Tobago* by C.R. Ottley; Lloyd Williams, N.I.C.A. Kingston; Virginia Turner, *The Jamaican Weekly Gleaner* (North American edition); Lizard Loebman, *Reggae Report;* Dawad Phillip, *The Daily Challenge;* Dr. Carlos Russell and Toni Hinton; Mali Olatunji; Ben Mapp; Julian Dibbell; and Donna Minkowitz.

The Names on the Board
An Ohio Teacher Dares Students to Envision a New Community
Jamie Rhein

The original lesson plan for my 11th grade American literature class was straightforward enough. Following a discussion of the Transcendentalists and utopian societies and after reading excerpts of Emerson's essay "Nature," the students were to break into groups and design their own utopias. Since this was generally a cooperative and diligent class, I wasn't concerned about leaving Friday morning's lesson in the hands of a substitute. That afternoon, as I read the substitute's note, I felt sick. She reported that most groups did well, but one group of boys could not move past the point of wondering what to do with gays.

I pictured the boys—boys I adored. They are the type of students who smile when they see you and gesture exuberantly in trying to get your attention. They are thrilled that you're their teacher, and, as I found out, they are anti-gay.

Besides being faced once more with the reality that my idea of a perfect world is a long way off, I found my sense of well-being for myself and those I love threatened. Not by some unknown force, but by young men I wanted to continue to like.

The "gay issue" is not one that I feel safe discussing in a classroom. My emotions run too high. I have a gay brother whom I love dearly. When students make any type of homophobic remarks, my usual response is to squelch the issue by explaining that such comments "aren't allowed." This time I wasn't there to stop the rumblings. This time, I realized, my continuing silence on the issue was unacceptable.

Monday morning, I knew I had to speak up. I feared that I was about to ruin my week, along with the good impression my students had of me, and open myself to hostile reactions from parents (and, soon after, administrators). I decided my brother's dignity was worth the risk of making a few waves. I greeted the class: "How was your weekend? Before we go any further with today's lesson, we need to deal with something that has been troubling me all weekend."

111

I told them I wasn't sure what to do about the matter. Then I turned to the board and began to write names: Jeff, Eric, Jerry, Cathy, Larry, Huck, Jeff . . .

"You already wrote 'Jeff,'" someone called out.

"There are two Jeffs," I said.

After writing about 20 names, I began to put stars by some of them.

"The ones with stars must be special," a student said. I nodded.

By this time, the class was silent, intent on my intentions. When my list was complete and I was ready to face the students, I turned around. "The names on the board are people I know and love. They are friends of mine, and they are gay.

"The stars are for ones who have AIDS or who have already died. One of them is my brother. One star is next to a person who cut my hair for eight years. He won't be cutting my hair any more because last summer someone who did not like gay people killed him. My friend would never have hurt anybody. He was one of the nicest, most gentle people you could ever know. More hate crimes are committed against gay people in this country than against any other group except African Americans.

"In my mind, a utopian society is one where everyone belongs. I don't care if you think it's wrong for someone to be gay. Or if you don't like gay people. I can promise you that someone in this class may be gay or have a gay relative or a gay friend. If you say that homosexuals should be excluded from society, or call someone a 'fag,' you will hurt someone. You will hurt me. No one has the right to hurt another human being. None of these people whose names are on the board would hurt anyone. That's all I want to say about it. There will be no discussion."

Everyone was listening. No one said a word. This was not the time for me to debate gay issues or to hear student viewpoints. I already knew some of them anyway. I wasn't interested in hearing if their opinions had changed. All I wanted was to get the sick feeling out of my soul and to let these students know that sometimes what is said in class does touch on the personal and sometimes the teacher does need to speak from the heart.

Emerson speaks of an ideal society where individuals respond to the world around them without egotism. I have discovered in teaching that egotism can serve a larger purpose. Sometimes, by offering the guidance of our unique personal perspectives, we can help students expand their own visions of Utopia.

Educators Protest Limits on Multicultural Mandate

Paula Ressler

V ery often people in universities feel insulated from the outside world by the heaviness of our work loads and our immersion in our teaching and research, but every so often an issue inserts itself that even the most insulated of us cannot ignore. When the Board of Education decided to take another stab at weakening multicultural education in this city, members of the Department of Teaching and Learning at New York University felt that we needed to respond. We have had many conversations that have increased our awareness about the issues and are continuing to look deeply into how these concerns affect us as educators.

On March 22, our collaboration resulted in a letter to the editor of the *New York Times*. Copies were also sent to Chancellor Ramon Cortines of the New York City Schools, Board of Education members and Mayor Rudolph Giuliani, among many others. Among faculty and teaching fellows signing this letter were LEARN members Becca Chase, John Mayher, Karen Ogulnick, Gordon Pradl, Paula Ressler, Sharon Shelton-Colangelo, Marilyn Sobelman and Harold Vine. It is our hope that if more people in education speak out, at some point this decision might be reversed and further efforts to erode multicultural education in this city will be halted. The letter reads as follows:

Open Letter to the Board of Education of the City of New York

On March 15, 1995, the Board of Education voted to limit the multicultural mandate for New York City public schools to only racial, ethnic and linguistic minorities, and to separate multiculturalism from anti-discrimination education. Since then, members of the Department of Teaching and Learning in the School of Education at New York University have been discussing this decision. At this time we wish to voice our deep concern publicly.

We feel that excluding issues such as disability, age, religion, gender and sexual orientation significantly weakens the multicultural mandate of our city's public schools. Furthermore, we feel that the decision to limit the multicultural mandate is designed primarily to placate a small but vocal group of people who wish to exclude lesbian and gay people from the multicultural curriculum and who refuse to accept that lesbians and gay men and youth and their families do indeed exist, attend schools, parent children, live and work in this city. Furthermore, they are entitled to the same respect accorded everyone else. We strongly urge the Board to reverse this damaging decision.

This decision will not only hurt lesbian and gay people, their relatives and friends, all of whom already experience tremendous discrimination in our society, but will hurt all groups in the city who face discrimination, whether because of race, religion, gender, age or ability. These divide-and-conquer tactics are designed to weaken the movement for equal, quality education for all by pitting one group against another at a time when our only hope is to work together to fight devastating and life-threatening budget cuts in education and human services. These include national and local budget cuts in programs affecting poor women, children, people with disabilities and the elderly; cuts in school lunch, transportation and bilingual education programs; and reversal of affirmative action legislation and legal protections for groups who have faced discrimination. Attorney General Vacco's decision to rescind employment rights to gay people in his own office, rights that have been in effect for the past fifteen years, is one example of such discrimination.

We do not believe that the Board's decision is designed to strengthen multicultural education and promote group tolerance as Board President Carol Gresser contends (NYT, editorial, 2/15/95). Excluding some groups from the curriculum weakens the essence of multiculturalism which is designed to help our children understand differences and appreciate one another. We also do not believe that the Board's decision will lead to more effective anti-discrimination education. Separating multicultural from anti-discrimination education makes a complete farce of the concept of multiculturalism, substituting superficial study for a deep exploration of the complexity of peoples, cultures, and their interrelationships, which only an inclusive view of multiculturalism can promote. If our department is to continue to educate reasonable, dedicated and caring teachers, we cannot embrace an educational policy that sanctions exclusion. Whether or not the Board continues to bow to political maneuvering, we will continue to provide an educational experience founded on inclusiveness, one that strengthens the voice of understanding and compassion in the schools of this city and throughout the country.

Sincerely, Faculty and Teaching Fellows Department of Teaching and Learning School of Education New York University

LEARN is a non-profit, tax exempt educational organization. P.O. Box 8103 FDR Station, New York, NY 10150.

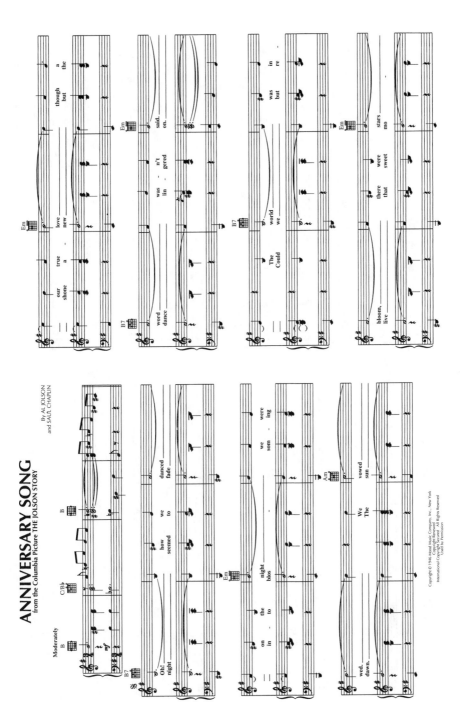

ANNIVERSARY SONG

from the Columbia Picture THE JOLSON STORY

By AL JOLSON
and SAUL CHAPLIN

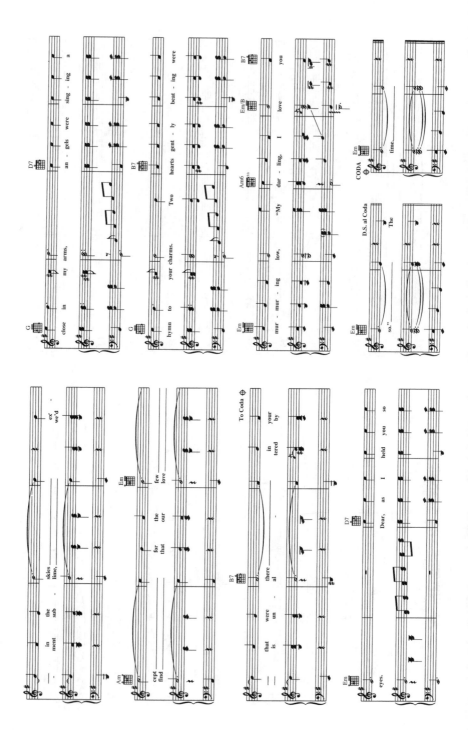

116

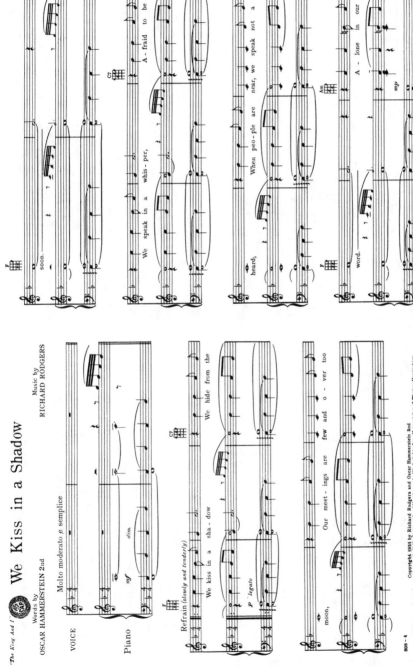
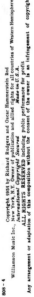

117

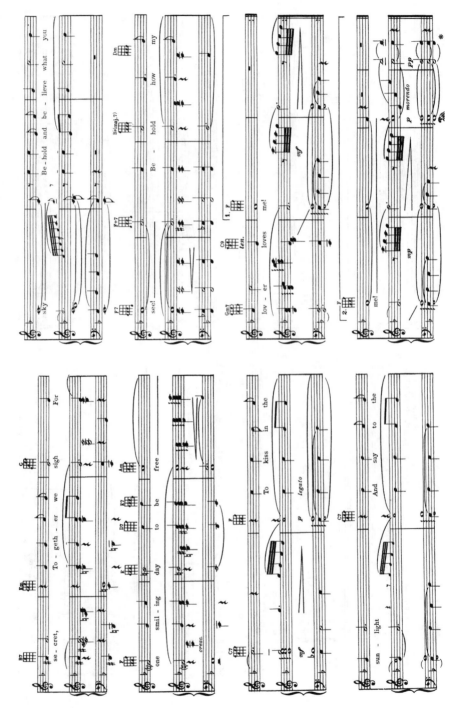

Bibliography

Associated Press. 1996. "$900,000 Won by Gay Man in Abuse Case." *The New York Times.* 21 November.

Aucoin, Don & Dabilis, Andy. 1992. "Jeers, Threats Greet Gays in South Boston Parade." *Boston Globe,* 16 March, pp. 1, 14.

Barnes, Douglas. 1976/1992. *From Communication to Curriculum.* 2d ed. Portsmouth, NH: Boynton/Cook.

Bass, Ellen & Kaufman, Kate. 1996. *Free Your Mind: The Book for Gay, Lesbian and Bisexual Youth—and Their Allies.* New York: Harper Perennial.

Blumenfeld, Warren J., ed. 1992. *Homophobia: How We All Pay the Price.* Boston: Beacon.

Blumenfeld, Warren J. & Lindop, Laurie. 1995. *Gay/Straight Alliances: A Student Guide.* Massachusetts Department of Education, Safe Schools Program for Gay and Lesbian Students.

Blumenfeld, Warren J. & Raymond, Diane. 1988. *Looking at Gay and Lesbian Life.* Boston: Beacon.

Boal, Augusto. 1974/1985. *Theatre of the Oppressed.* Trans. Charles A. & Maria-Odilia Leal McBride. New York: Theatre Communications Group.

———. 1992. *Games for Actors and Non-Actors.* Trans. Adrian Jackson. New York: Routledge.

Bolton, Gavin. 1992a. Workshop. London, U.K.: New York University, School of Education, Program in Educational Theatre—Study Abroad. Holborn Centre for Performing Arts. 27 July.

———. 1992b. *New Perspectives on Classroom Drama.* Hemel Hempstead, U.K.: Simon & Schuster Education.

Bozett, Frederick W. & Sussman, Marvin B. 1990. *Homosexuality and Family Relations.* New York: Harrington Park.

Britton, James. 1982. *Prospect and Retrospect: Selected Essays of James Britton.* Ed. Gordon Pradl. Montclair, NJ: Boynton/Cook.

Buckel, David. 1999. "Youth Bring Gay Rights Movement to School." *Lambda Update.* Lambda Legal Defense and Education Fund.

Chekhov, Michael. 1953. *To the Actor: On the Technique of Acting.* New York: Harper & Row.

Christen, Lesley. 1992. *Drama Skills for Life: A Handbook for Secondary Teachers.* Portsmouth, NH: Heinemann.

Cohen, Robert. 1978. *Acting Power.* Mountain View, CA: Mayfield.
————. 1984. *Acting One.* Mountain View, CA: Mayfield.
Courtney, Richard. 1980. *The Dramatic Curriculum.* New York: Drama Book Specialists.
December 2000. *Supporting Youth: Their Education and Survival.* New York: In the Life.
DeGeneres, Betty. 1999. *Love, Ellen: A Mother/Daughter Journey.* New York: Rob Weisback.
Dewey, John. 1900/1990. *The School and Society/The Child and the Curriculum.* Chicago: The University of Chicago Press.
Dixon, John. 1975. *Growth Through English: Set in the Perspective of the Seventies.* New York: Oxford University Press.
Douglas, Ann. 1999. "All Singing! All Dancing! All Gotham!" *The New York Times.* 28 May.
Ellsworth, Elizabeth. 1997. *Teaching Positions: Difference, Pedagogy, and the Power of Address.* New York: Teachers College.
Emunah, Renee. 1994. *Acting for Real: Drama Therapy Process, Technique, and Performance.* New York: Brunner/Mazel.
Epstein, Debbie, ed. 1994. *Challenging Lesbian and Gay Inequalities in Education.* Buckingham, England: Open University Press.
Errington, Edward. 1992. *Towards a Socially Critical Drama Education.* Victoria, Australia: Deakin University.
————. 1996. "Some Reflections on Researching Drama Classrooms." *Research in Drama Education* 1 (1): 23–32.
Ewen, Frederic. 1967. *Bertolt Brecht, His Life, His Art, and His Times.* New York: Citadel.
Feinberg, Leslie. 1997. *Transgender Warriors.* Boston: Beacon.
Fisher, Berenice. 1987. "The Heart Has Its Reasons: Feeling, Thinking and Community-Building in Feminist Education." *Women's Studies Quarterly* 15 (3&4): 47–58.
Freire, Paulo. 1970/1993. *Pedagogy of the Oppressed.* Trans. M. B. Ramos. New York: Continuum.
Fricke, Aaron. 1981. *Reflections of a Rock Lobster: A Story About Growing Up Gay.* Boston: Alyson.
Friend, Richard A. 1993. "Choices, Not Closets: Heterosexism and Homophobia in Schools." In *Beyond Silenced Voices: Class, Race, and Gender in United States Schools,* ed. Lois Weis and Michele Fine, 209–235. Albany: State University of New York.
Fuss, Diana. 1989. *Essentially Speaking: Feminism, Nature and Difference.* New York: Routledge.

Gardner, Howard. 1983/1985. *Frames of Mind: The Theory of Multiple Intelligences*. New York: Basic.
———. 1993. *Multiple Intelligences: The Theory in Practice*. New York: Basic.
———. 1995. "Reflections on Multiple Intelligences: Myths and Messages." *Phi Delta Kappan* (November): 200–209.
Gay and Lesbian Parents Association. 1996. *Both My Mom's Names Are Judy.* Video. San Francisco: Gay and Lesbian Parents Association.
"Gay Rights in California." 1999. Editorial. *The New York Times.* 6 October.
Gordon, Lenore. 1983. "What Do We Say When We Hear 'Faggot'?" *Interracial Books for Children Bulletin 14:* 25–27.
Griffin, Pat. 1992. "From Hiding Out to Coming Out: Empowering Lesbian and Gay Educators." In *Coming Out of the Classroom Closet: Gay and Lesbian Students, Teachers and Curricula,* ed. Karen M. Harbeck, 167–96. New York: Harrington Park.
Halliday, Michael A. K. 1989. *Spoken and Written Language.* 2d ed. Oxford: Oxford University Press.
Harbeck, Karen M., ed. 1992. *Coming Out of the Classroom Closet: Gay and Lesbian Students, Teachers and Curricula.* Binghamton, NY: Harrington Park.
Heathcote, Dorothy. 1984. *Dorothy Heathcote: Collected Writings on Education and Drama.* Ed. Liz Johnson and Cecily O'Neill. Evanston, IL: Northwestern University Press.
Heathcote, Dorothy & Bolton, Gavin. 1995. *Drama for Learning: Dorothy Heathcote's Mantle of the Expert Approach to Education.* Portsmouth, NH: Heinemann.
Herdt, Gilbert, ed. 1989. *Gay and Lesbian Youth.* New York: Harrington Park.
Heron, Ann, ed. 1995. *Two Teenagers in Twenty: Writings by Gay and Lesbian Youth.* Boston: Alyson.
Holden, Stephen. 1999. "Though Rodgers, Thou Hart, So Fuzzy, So Smart." *The New York Times.* 6 January.
Homes, A. M. 1989. *Jack.* New York: Vintage.
Howey, Noelle & Samuels, Ellen. 2000. *Out of the Ordinary: Growing Up with Gay, Lesbian and Transgender Parents.* New York: St. Martins.
Hunter, Joyce. 1990. "Violence Against Lesbian and Gay Male Youths." *Journal of Interpersonal Violence 5* (3): 295–300.
Hunter, Joyce & Schaecher, Robert. 1987. "Stresses on Lesbian and Gay Adolescents in Schools." *Social Work in Education 9* (3): 180–89.
Intersex Society of North America (ISNA). 1996. *www.isna.org.*
Jackson, Tony, ed. 1993. *Learning through Theatre: New Perspectives on Theatre-in-Education.* London: Routledge.

Jennings, Kevin, ed. 1994. *One Teacher in 10: Gay and Lesbian Educators Tell Their Stories*. Boston: Alyson.

Jennings, Sue. 1995. *Dramatherapy with Children and Adolescents*. London: Routledge.

Johnson, David Read. 1981. "Some Diagnostic Implications of Drama Therapy." In *Drama in Therapy, Volume Two: Adults*, ed. Gertrud Schattner and Richard Courtney, 13–34. New York: Drama Books.

Jolson, Al & Chaplin, Saul. 1946. "Anniversary Song." Based on 1880 waltz "Danube Waves," by J. Ivanovici. Milwaukee, WI: Hal Leonard.

Khayatt, Madiha Didi. 1992. *Lesbian Teachers: An Invisible Presence*. Albany: State University of New York.

Landy, Robert J. (1986). *Drama Therapy: Concepts and Practices*. Springfield, MA: Charles C. Thomas.

———. 1993. *Persona and Performance: The Meaning of Role in Drama, Therapy, and Everyday Life*. New York: Guilford.

Lipkin, Arthur. (1999). *Understanding Homosexuality, Changing Schools: A Text For Teachers, Counselors, and Administrators*. Boulder, CO: Westview.

McCaslin, Nellie. 1990. *Creative Drama in the Classroom*. New York: Longman.

Meisner, Sanford. 1987. *On Acting*. New York: Vintage.

Miller, D. A. 1998. *Place for Us: Essay on the Broadway Musical*. Cambridge: Harvard University Press.

Moffett, James & Wagner, Betty Jane. 1973/1976. *Student-Centered Language Arts and Reading, K-13: A Handbook for Teachers*. 2nd ed. Boston: Houghton Mifflin.

Namaste, Viviane K. 2000. *Invisible Lives: The Erasure of Transsexual and Transgendered People*. Chicago: University of Chicago Press.

Neelands, Jonothan. 1984. *Making Sense of Drama: A Guide to Classroom Practice*. London: Heinemann.

———. 1990. *Structuring Drama Work*. Cambridge: Cambridge University Press.

Nieves, Evelyn. 1990. "Attacks on a Gay Teen-Ager Prompt Outrage and Soul-Searching." *The New York Times*. 19 February A1+.

Noel, Peter, with Marriott, Robert. 1993. "Batty Boys in Babylon: Can Gay West Indians Survive the 'Boom Bye Bye' Posses?" *The Village Voice*, 38 (2): 29–39.

O'Neill, Cecily. 1995. *Drama Worlds: A Framework for Process Drama*. Portsmouth, NH: Heinemann.

O'Neill, Cecily & Lambert, Alan. 1988. *Drama Structures*. London: Hutchinson Education.

Owens, Robert E. 1998. *Queer Kids*. New York: Harrington Park.

Parmeter, Sarah-Hope & Reti, Irene, eds. 1988. *The Lesbian in Front of the Classroom: Writings by Lesbian Teachers*. Santa Cruz: HerBooks.

Pharr, Suzanne. 1988. *Homophobia: A Weapon of Sexism*. Little Rock: Chardon.

Piaget, Jean. 1964/1967. *Six Psychological Studies*. Trans. Anita Tenzer. New York: Random House.

Pradl, Gordon M., ed. 1982. *Prospect and Retrospect: Selected Essays of James Britton*. Montclair, NJ: Boynton/Cook.

Rabinovitz, Jonathan. 1998. "A School is Split Over Boys in Skirts." *The New York Times*. 3 April: B1.

Remafedi, Gary. 1994. *Death by Denial: Studies of Suicide in Gay and Lesbian Teenagers*. Boston: Alyson.

Ressler, Paula. 1995. "Educators Protest Limits on Multicultural Mandate." *LEARN*. June.

Rhein, Jamie. 1998. "The Names on the Board: An Ohio Teacher Dares Students to Envision a New Community." *Teaching Tolerance* (Spring): 62–63.

Robson, Ruthann. 1998. *Sappho Goes to Law School*. New York: Columbia.

Rodgers, Richard (music), & Hammerstein, Oscar II (book and lyrics). 1951. "We Kiss in a Shadow." From *The King and I*, musical play based on *Anna and the King of Siam*, by Margaret Landon. Milwaukee, WI: Hal Leonard.

Rogers, Carl R. 1961. *On Becoming a Person: A Therapist's View of Psychotherapy*. Boston: Houghton Mifflin.

———. 1980/1995. *A Way of Being*. Boston: Houghton Mifflin.

Romesburg, Don. 1996. *Young, Gay, and Proud*. 4th ed. Boston: Alyson.

Ryan, Caitlin & Futterman, Donna. 1999. *Lesbian and Gay Youth: Care and Counseling*. New York: Columbia University Press.

Savin-Williams, Ritch C. 1992. Deadly Silence: Our Neglect of Lesbian, Gay Male, and Bisexual Youths. Prepared for the APA CLGC/CYF Subcommittee on Lesbian, Gay and Bisexual Youths.

Schutzman, Mady & Cohen-Cruz, Jan, eds. 1994. *Playing Boal: Theatre, Therapy, Activism*. London: Routledge.

Scotta, Carole (prod.) & Berliner, Alain (dir.). 1997. *Ma Vie en Rose (My Life in Pink)*. Film. Available from Sony Pictures Classics.

Sears, James T. 1991. *Growing Up Gay in the South: Race, Gender, and Journeys of the Spirit*. New York: Haworth.

———. 1992. "Educators, Homosexuality, and Homosexual Students: Are Personal Feelings Related to Professional Beliefs?" In *Coming Out of the Classroom Closet*, ed. Karen M. Harbeck, 29–79. New York: Harrington Park.

Slade, Peter. 1954. *Child Drama.* London: University of London Press.

Smith, Gwendolyn Ann. 1999, 2000. *Remembering Our Dead.* A Project of Gender Education and Advocacy, hosted by Above and Beyond. *www.gender.org/remember.*

Spolin, Viola. 1963/1983. *Improvisations for the Theater.* Evanston, IL: Northwestern University Press.

————. 1986. *Theater Games for the Classroom: A Teacher's Handbook.* Evanston, IL: Northwestern University Press.

Sullivan, Andrew, ed. 1997. *Same-Sex Marriage: Pro and Con—A Reader.* New York: Vintage.

Telljohann, Susan K., Price, James H., Poureslami, Mohammad & Easton, Alyssa. 1995. "Teaching About Sexual Orientation by Secondary Health Teachers." *Journal of School Health* 65 (1): 18–22.

Unks, Gerald, ed. 1995. *The Gay Teen: Educational Practice and Theory for Lesbian, Gay, and Bisexual Adolescents.* New York: Routledge.

Uribe, Virginia & Harbeck, Karen M. 1992. "Addressing the Needs of Lesbian, Gay, and Bisexual Youth: The Origins of PROJECT 10 and School-Based Intervention." In *Coming Out of the Classroom Closet,* ed. Karen M. Harbeck 9–28. New York: Harrington Park.

Vygotsky, L. S. 1915–1935/1978. *L. S. Vygotsky: Mind in Society: The Development of Higher Psychological Processes.* Ed. Michael Cole, Vera John-Steiner, Sylvia Scribner, & Ellen Souberman. Cambridge: Harvard University.

Walling, Donovan R., ed. 1996. *Open Lives, Safe Schools: Addressing Gay and Lesbian Issues in Education.* Bloomington, IN: Phi Delta Kappa Educational Foundation.

Way, Brian. 1972. *Development Through Drama.* New York: Humanities.

Weiler, Kathleen. 1991. "Freire and a Feminist Pedagogy of Difference." *Harvard Educational Review.* 61 (4): 449–74.

Weis, Lois & Fine, Michelle, eds. 1993. *Beyond Silenced Voices: Class, Race, and Gender in United States Schools.* Albany: State University of New York Press.

Willen, Liz. 1994. "Rainbow Over: Watered-Down Version of Teachers Guide to Make Rounds." *New York Newsday* 15 February: 1.

Willett, John, ed. 1964. *Brecht on Theatre.* Frankfurt: Suhrkamp Verlag.

Woodman, Natalie Jane, ed. 1992. *Lesbian and Gay Lifestyles: A Guide for Counseling and Education.* New York: Irvington.

Woodson, Jacqueline. 1995. *From the Notebooks of Melanin Sun.* New York: Scholastic.

Woog, Dan. 1995. *School's Out: The Impact of Gay and Lesbian Issues on America's Schools.* Boston: Alyson.